BREAKING

FOOD

CHAINS

BREAKING
FOOD
CHAINS

A Personal Guide to Culinary Freedom

Shidaun "Africano" Campbell

On-Demand Publishing, LLC.
Scotts Valley, CA

Breaking Food Chains

Copyright © 2016 Shidaun Campbell

All rights reserved.

Published by On-Demand Publishing, LLC. 2016

Scotts Valley, CA, USA

First Printing, 2016

ISBN 978-1537171388

No parts of this publication may be reproduced, stored in a retrieval system, or transmitted in any form or by any means, electronic, mechanical, photocopying, recording, or otherwise, without the prior written permission of the copyright owner.

This book is sold subject to the condition that it shall not, by way of trade or otherwise, be lent, resold, hired out, or otherwise circulated without the publisher's prior consent in any form of binding or cover other than that in which it is published and without a similar condition including this condition being imposed on the subsequent purchaser. Under no circumstances may any part of this book be photocopied for resale.

Cover Photography from iStockPhoto.com

DEDICATED TO:

- Grandpa Narome
- Stanley Jr.
- Dewan

And all the others who left us too soon....

TABLE OF CONTENTS

PART I
Building Blocks:
What you need to know first

A Chance to Heal	3
You Are What You Think *Toxic words to eliminate from your vocabulary*	5
What's Eating You? *Understanding emotional eating*	11
The 5 Steps to Curing Emotional Eating	15
Food Is Energy	19
Mood Foods *Improving your mood with the right foods*	21
Deficiencies and Supplements *Ending cravings with proper nutrition*	23
The Eating Lifestyle Cycle *Understanding the bigger picture*	25
The Façade of Losing Weight *Never count calories again!*	29
A Numbers Game *How eating right can save us money*	31
Location, Location, Location *Food's connection to our ancestry*	33

The Cultural and Social Kick   35
Eating well without sacrificing your social life

Non-GMO and Organic   37
Why the hype?

Inflammatory and Mucus-Causing Foods   41
Combating chronic inflammation

Alkaline vs. Acid Forming Foods   45
No longer be prone to disease

Alkaline Water   49

Water Therapy   53
The dehydration cure

Edible Foods   57
Why more is not always better

Food Combining   59
The indigestion cure

Eating in Season   65
Getting the most out of your food

Know Your Body   83
Understanding the digestive process

Disease Explained   87
The true definition of disease

Common Food-Related Diseases   89
A comprehensive list

PART II
Culinary Bondage:
What foods are keeping us down + their healthy alternatives

Corn	95
Wheat	97
Pasta	101
Soy	103
Red Meat	105
White Meat	107
Halal & Kosher Options	109
Fish	113
Smoked Foods	115
Rice	117
Sugar	119
Honey	123
Eggs	125
Fried Foods	127
Salty Snacks	129
Dairy	131
Caffeine	135
Coffee	137
Carbonated Beverages	139
White Potatoes	141
Bananas	143
Pasteurized Juice	145
Tap Water	147
Canned Foods	149
Artificial Ingredients	151
"But, It's Natural!"	153
Cooking Oils	155
Fast Food	159
Peanuts	161
Breath Fresheners	163
Alcoholic Beverages	165
Dried Fruit	167
Seasonings & Spices	169

Reading Labels 171
What to keep in mind when shopping around

Processed and Overcooked Foods 173
How to get the most out of your food

Breakfast Foods 177
The right way to start your day

PART III
Action:
Putting the knowledge into practice

Breakin' It Down: Soaking and Sprouting 181
Iron deficiency stops here

The Bean Dilemma 183
How to cook beans the right way

Fermenting Foods 185
Boosting digestion and immune health

Candida Overgrowth 189
The cause of many diseases

Nutritional Yeast 181
Good or bad?

Allergies and Intolerances 193
Getting to the root of allergic reactions

The Ultimate Four 195
Key things to remember

Freedom Foods 197
Everything you can eat

Recipes

Millet Grits	201
Sweet & Spicy Quinoa	202
Buckwheat Couscous	204
Amaranth Porridge	205
Avocado Salad	207
Beet Salad	208
Savory Oatmeal	209
Curried Red Lentil Soup	210
Popcorn-Style Rice Cakes	211
Savory Sweet Potatoes	212
Oven Fried Okra	213

What's in Your Toolbox?   215
A few things to invest in & why

Protein Is Overrated   217
Why your protein shake may be unnecessary

The Replacement Diet   223
Don't waste it, replace it!

The "Lose It" List   225
How to create your personal action plan

Fasting   229
Reboot your tastebuds

Cleanses and Detox Programs   231
When to go on one and how

Listening to Your Body   233

It's a Process, Not a Diet   235
Honoring every step of the way

Living Situations   239
Eating well no matter where you live

Microwaves   241
   More than a quick fix

Occupational Hazard   243
   Eating well no matter where your work

Eating Out   245
   How to find healthy food on the go

Shopping Around   247
   Where to get good food

The "Food Desert" Epidemic   249

QUICK REFERENCE CHARTS

Words to Replace	9
Alkaline Foods	48
pH Levels	50
Fruit Categories	62
Proper Food Combinations	64
Seasonal Fruits (U.S)	80
Seasonal Vegetables (U.S.)	81
The Digestive System	84
Common Food-Related Diseases	89
Freedom Foods	198
Recommended Daily Protein Intake (Formula)	220

SPECIAL THANKS TO:

- Mom
- Dad
- Soumayah
- Queen Afua
- Saa'Shalom
- Femi

And everyone else who gave me nuggets of wisdom and inspiration along my journey.

Preface

Generational illness and diseases that "run in the family" stem from unhealthy lifestyles and thought patterns. These range from heart attack, stroke to cancer and anemia. One of the ways we can break this cycle is by changing what and how we eat. By doing this, we are empowered to reverse these supposed "genetic" diseases and end the cycle of suffering for generations to come.

Do you want to leave a legacy? Do you want to live long enough to see it and be healthy enough to enjoy it? You are going to have to give up a lot of those things you "love" because you love and value your body, your health, your life and your family more. Most likely, you will learn to love some new things along the way. Trust me, your body will love you back.

Did you know that eating well is a form of self-love? When those we care about are out of line, sometimes, we have to give them "tough love." You care about yourself, right? If you, in any way, feel that your body is out of line, maybe it's time to give yourself some tough love. If you do not, who else will? This book will not tell you everything but it will give you the basics to keep learning. There is a lot of information out there and once you start learning, it will be hard to stop.

My Story...

I wrote this book because I am tired of watching people in my family die or struggle with disease and feeling I could do nothing about it. I am half Iranian and African American. On my African-American side of my family, too many of my loved ones have died young and battled with heart disease, obesity, and cancer. On my Iranian side, many of the women in my family have suffered from digestive problems and fibroids. Before I was born (while my mother was still carrying me), this almost claimed my life, as one of my mother's fibroids fought with me for nutrients while I was in the womb. In order to keep me from dying, she had to get a C-section and I was born prematurely.

I was diagnosed with asthma before the age of two. Being premature, my lungs were undeveloped and asthma ran in both sides of my family. I began having bouts with severe eczema as a child and found out that I was allergic to all things dairy (milk, cheese, etc.) at the age of eight. I was also allergic to a multitude of other things including dogs, cats, dust, pollen, food coloring and artificial preservatives. If you could name it, then I was probably allergic to it! At this point, some of you would say "Oh, well, it sounds like you had no choice but to eat healthy." Everyone has a choice, even if they are knowingly undermining their own health. I simply chose not to get sick by eating and being around certain things I knew would make me feel bad. Have you seen an asthmatic who smokes cigarettes or someone who is overweight in the all-you-can-eat-buffet-line? I have. I would ask myself why they would do that to themselves and I realized that they simply made a choice. This time, it was to the detriment of their health.

In college, I had an extreme breakout of eczema. I was covered in rashes from head to toe. The incessant itching and burning made it almost impossible to sleep and made it difficult to enjoy watching TV or dancing. Things that I would usually do for fun became tasks. Have you ever experienced something that took the light out of your everyday life? I did, and it was like having the chicken-pox for two months. Imagine how many of us are actually experiencing some form of everyday discomfort or dis-ease and we simply normalize it (make it the norm). Although we are not paying attention to these things, they are playing in the background and affecting our everyday experiences more than we think. Everything we put off for later, put in the background, throw under the rug or shove away in a vault eventually surfaces. Usually, the longer it is hidden, the more difficult and detrimental it can become. Eventually, we have to face the music. So, I did what any person would do. I went to the doctor. This so-called-doctor actually looked at my skin, went on his computer, did a search on Google (in front of me), and proceeded to diagnose me with Scabies. He ended his statement with "...but I'm not sure." Then, he dismissed me and gave me a prescribed bottle of antibiotics. I was baffled.

Keep in mind that I was raised by my mother, a dietitian, nutritionist and homeopathic doctor, as well as my father, a health-conscious musician and aspiring chef. However, neither my parents nor my doctor could fix my so-called problem. I had finally hit rock bottom and hit my breaking point. At this point, I needed to know if it was anything I was eating. Though I was avoiding all of my food allergies, I was not sure. Extreme circumstances call for extreme measures. Consequently, I took everything out of my diet and started from scratch, only eating basmati rice with sea salt for three days. Then, every three days, I would add an ingredient. By the end of the first week, I was eating beans and rice with salt and pepper (much better than a bland bowl of white rice). By the end of the second week, I was eating black bean soup with carrots and celery, cream of rice for breakfast and an avocado salad for lunch. Within two weeks, my Eczema was basically non-existent! This was huge considering doctors told me my eczema was incurable, but I was curing it simply by removing things from my diet.

I continued this plan for 6 months and every time I reacted to an added ingredient (in any way), I knew exactly what it was and I would simply add it to the "Lose It" list. I also switched out my lotions for shea butter, my body sprays to essential oils and started getting more sun. All of these things (and more) have helped me treat my eczema and asthma as well as boosted my energy level over the years. After almost 10 years, I am now writing this book and saving everyone the trouble of eating salty rice for a week. Through my research, I have come to realize that we are not different. Research shows that everything that I had on my "Do Not Eat" list are things that are simply harmful to the human body and contribute to a multitude of diseases, disorders, illnesses and cancers. Generally, most of us do not see these problems show up until later. However, due to my heightened sensitivity, I was able to pinpoint what these ingredients were and eliminate them from my lifestyle before they became life-threatening.

If you are reading this book, I want you to know that this is not out of reach. You do not have to be some amazing chef or health guru to eat well. All you need is the patience to learn and the desire to change your lifestyle. If you are tired of seeing yourself and those around you suffer, this book is dedicated to *you*.

MEDICAL DISCLAIMER:

This book is not intended to be a substitute for the medical advice of a licensed physician. The reader should consult with their doctor in any matters relating to his/her health and particularly with respect to any symptoms that may require diagnosis or medical attention.

PART I

Building Blocks

What you need to know first

2

A Chance to Heal

Did you know that the body can completely heal itself if it is given the chance? Just like a flower can be chopped down or trimmed and still grow back just as beautiful weeks later. Though it may take more than a few weeks, our bodies have the natural ability to heal themselves over time. Now, imagine if that flower is covered in thick, black oil. Do you think it would grow back or would it wither away and die? Of course, cars run off of oil (petroleum to be exact) but flowers are not cars. So why will a flower not thrive in this situation? The same rule applies to our bodies. When we bog down our bodies with the wrong things, we limit its ability to heal itself. However, when we take care of our bodies, our bodies take care of us. It is able to run smoothly, like a well-oiled machine, and lives up to its full potential. Flowers need water and nutrient-rich soil as much as our bodies need fresh water and nutrient-rich, plant based foods to thrive and regenerate. If we give our bodies a chance to live up to its full potential we may be surprised at what it can actually do. With a cleaner diet, we will realize that even our bodies smell better; even when we sweat. I am not saying to completely ditch deodorant, but you may not need as much as often.

I wrote this book for the everyday person. This is not a scientific journal, or a dissertation of any sorts. The information provided is based on my personal experiences, research and observances from over 10 years as a health practitioner. If there is any skepticism at any point, consult a professional or simply research the information provided in this text. The purpose of this book is to serve as a guide to healthier living, so that we as a people can heal.

WORDS OF WISDOM

Ever look at a baby?

They know exactly when they are hungry, stop eating when they are full, and only eat what agrees with them. Not to mention, almost as soon as they eat, the excess waste is moving out of their bodies. Everything is new and is looked at with a sense of wonderment in a baby's eyes. Colors are brighter and smiles are bigger. As we get older, we let our minds and habits get in the way of our enjoyment of life. Our goal is to get back to what it is like to be a baby. To give our bodies, hearts and minds a fresh start. And this happens one step at a time.

You Are What You Think

Toxic words to eliminate from your vocabulary

We all know the phrase "you are what you eat," but what about our thoughts? Do we have to think before we act? If that is the case, and eating is an action, then maybe, just maybe, we should give our thoughts and words more credit. The reality is that our thoughts create words and our words create our reality. Before we start eliminating things from our lifestyle, we should start by eliminating a few key toxic words. These words can stop you in your tracks and halt your progress. They can even be emotional triggers that make us want to eat various unhealthy things. When we feel the need to say these words, mentally and verbally it is important to replace them with a better word or phrase.

Can't - *"I can't eat that." "I can't stop smoking." "I can't live without sweets".*

Using this word takes the power away from us and gives it away to someone or something else. As if we do not have a choice. Everything is a choice. Even when we feel these choices are limited, we choose from those limited choices and even choose to believe we are limited in these choices. The reality is that there is always another option. When we say, "I can't" we are really telling ourselves, "I had no choice" and, in turn, giving away our power and the ability to choose. We choose what we believe and believe what we choose. Believing that you cannot is a choice and so is believing in yourself. Replace this word with "I choose to" and watch your perspective change. "I choose to not eat that (because I know it'll make me feel bad)", "I choose to not stop smoking", "I choose not to live without sweets". If we are doing something and are not getting the outcome we want, we simply say, "I am working on it." This leaves room for progress as opposed to simply cutting off the possibility of being able to do it at all.

Sorry - *"I'm sorry for breaking my diet."*

The word "sorry" is synonymous with the words "poor" and "pitiful". So, when we say, "I'm sorry", we are also telling ourselves, "I'm poor and pitiful." This is another one of those words that takes the power away from you and makes you the victim. It is one thing to accept where we were at a certain point in a process. It is another thing to wallow in it. Granted, it is helpful to admit when we are wrong (especially in a relationship).

Anytime we feel ourselves needing to apologize with "I'm sorry", we instead can tell ourselves, "I honor where I am" (in the process). By honoring (respecting), where you were (in regards to what you feel the need to apologize for), you are able to look at what you are thinking and how you felt when you did what made you feel the need to apologize. By doing this, we are not putting ourselves down but making the change to not do the act again (unless you choose to). Every time we trip up or fall, it is an opportunity to learn more about ourselves, become stronger and eventually become that person we have always wanted to look up to. Be unapologetically who we are. Make our weaknesses our strengths and our strengths our superpowers. All of us are 100% responsible for our own health and well-being. When it comes down to a long-term life of wellness, no one else can heal us, but *us*.

Problem - There is no such thing as a problem, just an opportunity for growth. Replace the word problem with the word "situation" or "test." Using these words help you look at these moments in a positive light as opposed to something that is simply a thorn in your side that you are annoyed by.

But - *"I want to eat better but..." "I could have more money but..."*

The use of the word "but" simply omits the possibility of another choice. It does this by giving power to something that truly does not have power and reinforces the negative. Saying, "I want to eat better but (I do not have enough money)", gives money power over your ability to eat better. Even though there are ways to eat well without hurting your wallet. Saying, "I could have more money but (I have too many bills)", gives the bills (and the entities sending them) power over our financial prosperity, as if they have direct access to your bank account and direct control over how much money we put in our piggy bank.

"But" is a gateway word to other negations (such as "can't"). We are not victims. We are creators of our own reality. Where there is a will, there is a way. Can we all think back to a time when we really needed or wanted something and we figured out a way to get it? If so, then we already understand this phrase firsthand. If not, then you have an opportunity to find out exactly what you are capable of. Either way, we might be surprised just how far we can go! Start replacing the word "but" with "however." This word represents a choice among options. We could be unhealthy, however, we are choosing to take control of our lives and take the first step today!

Do not - "Do not" represents your choice "not" to "do" something. So, whether we choose "not" to want something or "not" to understand something, remember that it is still a choice. Replace "I do not want" with "I am choosing (the better of the two options)" and Replace "I do not know/understand" with "I am learning (about)". This takes you from a position of complacency to forward movement.

Try - We often think and say things like, *"I will try to do it."* When we use the word try, we are telling ourselves that we are not fully committing to something. This stems from doubt and exhibits uncertainty. When you are not sure you can do something, you "try." Replace the word "try" with "give it my all" or "give it everything I've got." For example, replace "I will try to eat healthier" with "I will give it everything I've got to eat healthier." Say these out loud. Do you feel the difference? One speaks in uncertainty (which stems from fear) while the other invokes our spirit of determination. This allows us to succeed by facing whatever it is head on.

WORDS TO REPLACE

~~Can't~~ → "I choose not to..."

~~Sorry~~ → "I honor where I am"

~~Problem~~ → "Situation / Test"

~~But~~ → "However"

~~Don't~~ → "I am choosing not to..."

~~Try~~ → "I will give it my all"

10

What's Eating You?

Understanding emotional eating

Sweets - We crave sweets when we want to feel the "sweetness" of life. Often it is when our talents and abilities are not being put to use. Other times, we feel let down by something or someone and, in response to the harshness of life, we want something sweet and comforting. Ice cream is a choice vice for many of us because of its cool softness and sweetness. This is a great contrast to the harsh realities of life. Sadness, depression or simply feeling let down in any way (by ourselves or others) can drive us to eating sweets.

Now we must ask ourselves, do we really want sweets or do we simply want to feel loved and fulfilled? What is missing from our lives and how can we go about bringing the balance?

Salty Snacks - We often crave salt when our bodies are low on potassium. However, when we are craving something crunchy and salty, we are generally feeling anxious and do not even know it. There is a soothing effect to that "crunch" we crave. Think about it. When do we find ourselves eating a bag of chips or popcorn? Usually, it is when we are doing activities that require us to be still. Like, watching TV, movies, sports, working on a school project, studying or reading. Our bodies are still, but in our subconscious minds, we are going over a deadline coming up, how much money we have, problems in our relationships, etc.

We are mentally "crunching" away at our enjoyment of life while trying to keep our thoughts and worries at bay so that we can "relax." But, this is not true relaxation because we are not giving back to our bodies. True relaxation results in living with a balanced body and mind. And, if we are simply keeping our thoughts at bay, this does not allow us to sift through our thoughts and emotions to have a more resolute mind. So, the next time we crave something salty or crunchy, we must ask ourselves, "What is it that I am anxious or irritated about?"

Have you ever started eating a bag of chips, looked down a few minutes later and it was almost gone without you realizing it? We even do this when we are not hungry which tells me that it has more to do with how we feel than how hungry we are.

Overeating - We overeat when we feel unfulfilled. This can be in our profession, our relationships or anything in between. Take a moment and think about the word *fulfillment* and break it down. This begins with the verb fulfill. Breaking this word into two words, "Full" and "Fill," it begins to make sense when it comes to why we overeat. We eat to feel *full*. If we are not feeling whole or experiencing the *fullness* of life, then we will *fill* our stomachs in order to replicate that feeling.

What could you be doing to feed your spirit? Some of us jog, run, write, dance or teach. As a performing artist, once I began to get back on stage again, I stopped eating as much. I realized when I was satisfied and stopped eating. Though it was not every day, it gave me a sense of fulfillment. Even if it is for a fraction of your day, what is something that we could do that would make us feel whole or complete? Remember, it is not up to anyone but ourselves. We are in the driver's seat.

What about not having an appetite at all?
We eat to live. Not wanting to eat is often connected to a lack of desire to live. Perhaps we are tired of day-to-day life or simply feel we are undeserving of love and living. In some way, we have lost our appetite for life and this is what needs to be addressed. This is why there is always an emotional connection to not having an appetite. It also calls for the need to completely cleanse our bodies of waste, toxins, worms and parasites that may be affecting our appetite. These things suck the life out of us, including our zeal for life. When our bodies are deficient in minerals, this can also affect our appetite in a negative manner. Cleanse! We have to *give* our bodies the supplemental nutrients it needs and get to the root of the challenges that impact loss of appetite on an emotional level.

Eating Yourself to Sleep - Other than a need for discipline and healthy eating patterns, hunger is not the only reason we get the midnight munchies. When we wind down at night, we have to deal with our thoughts, and some of us do not like that. One way we combat this is by distracting ourselves with food. By eating ourselves to sleep, we do not have to deal with our thoughts.

But, this is only a temporary fix and thoughts will always be there. When you feel like eating late, we have to ask ourselves, "What thoughts or feelings am I trying to avoid right now?" Write them down in a journal to make them more tangible. Journal how we feel at the moment and why. Doing this helps us work through our feelings versus avoiding them. Our bodies and our hearts will thank us.

Knowing why we eat what we eat empowers us. Aside from vitamin and mineral deficiencies, these cravings are usually emotional. Every time we crave something sweet or crunchy, ask yourself, "What am I emotionally feeling right now?" "Is it anything other than happy and fulfilled?" The sooner we recognize the emotional reasons behind why we eat what we eat, the sooner we can address these things and start on a path to truly enjoying our lives (free of disease).

Think about it. With food, we are unconsciously self-medicating when it comes to our thoughts and emotions! Now, the question is, which medicine would we prefer? The one with the negative side effects that makes us feel bad later or the one that only makes us feel good. Eating and drinking things that rejuvenate our bodies balances not only our stomachs, but our emotions. When we are conscious of *why* we are eating what we are eating, we eat to live instead of live to eat. Foods that are good for us help us tackle these everyday thoughts and feelings that we are trying to avoid by feeding our bodies *and* brains.

With every bite and every sip, let us breathe life into our bodies. If what we are eating is not doing this, then we replace it with what will.

The 5 Steps to Cure Emotional Eating

Adjusting our diet is not only a physical process but an emotional one. We begin to clean up how we eat and how we feel simultaneously, which is why we call major shifts in our diet a *"cleansing process."* During a cleanse, we often crave something that we have removed from our diets. This is often due to the fact that what we were eating was used to remedy how we felt (e.g. anxious, frustrated, depressed, or unfulfilled). It is important to pay attention to when we are craving something because it is either connected to a nutritional deficiency or an emotional habit. Pinpointing when we have these cravings allows us to address how we feel and change how we cope with these feelings in ways that are healthy.

When we have a craving, we must ask ourselves:

"What emotion am I feeling right now?"
What am I holding onto from the past?"
"What is it that I need to let go of?"

Once we find out what that emotion is, what triggered it and what the root cause of it is, we will realize that it is connected to a specific event or person from the past. This is when we started coping in this way and we have had this habit ever since. "When did I start eating a bag of potato chips all by myself in one sitting?" "When did I begin eating a whole pint of ice cream during a movie?" "Was it after my first break up?" "Or when I got fired from my job years ago?" Asking ourselves questions like these are necessary to get to the root cause of emotional eating. We acknowledge that emotional eating is real. It is important to *own* it and recognize where we are and why. We also understand that how we feel affects how we eat and vice-versa. Once we have a grasp on the emotion we feel when we crave something and where it came from, we can continue along the steps to curing emotional eating:

1.) **Acknowledge** what/who it is and the role it played in our lives.
2.) **Separate** who we *are* from the experience we had. We are not our experiences. We only *learn* from them. We do not *become* them.
3.) **Meditate** journal, "ohm" it out, jog, dance, sing, go to therapy, speak to someone we trust. Let ourselves work though what it is that we want to change and how.
4.) **Release** whatever it is from our hearts and minds. Lighten the load by no longer taking ownership of it. It is not our burden to carry. Take the lesson and leave the rest.
5.) **Confront** the person or event that affected us for resolution and closure.

For many, step 5 is often the most intimidating part. On the other hand, once we get through step 4, it no longer seems as daunting since we have been able to release whatever we have felt and are ready for closure. This may involve confronting them physically or simply in your mind (e.g. writing a letter telling them how we feel and how what they did affected us. You may choose to store the letter in a safe space or burn it to represent the ending of a chapter in your life.) Revisiting this person, place or experience often shows us where we are in the process and if we still need more time to let go. Remember, *detachment is good, distance is not.* We do not distance ourselves from our emotions. We CONFRONT them by going through the 5 steps above so that we can heal and continue on our journey healthier and happier than we began.

WORDS OF WISDOM

Slow down!

Practice mindfulness. Taking your time while consciously chewing your food lets your brain register that your body is full. This will keep you from overeating. The key here is not to eat until we are full, but to eat until we are satisfied. Feeling "stuffed" may seem gratifying, but we end up being so tired because of it that it renders us completely useless for the next hour. It is important to give the body a break. It also improves digestion, which means we will get more nutrients out of our food. Trust me. Our bodies and our wallets will thank us.

Food Is Energy

Do we want our kids to have a more balanced level of energy and do better at their schoolwork? Would we like to have more energy and better focus at work? If so, we need to be even more aware of how and what we eat affects us on an energetic level!

Everything is energy, according to quantum physics. This energy can either be negative or positive. This means that something or someone can either give us energy or take it away. It can either make us feel alive or lethargic. Ever eaten something and walked away feeling drained? If so, this would mean that whatever we were eating was charged with negative energy. When we eat, this energy transfers from our food to our bodies. This is when the saying, "you are what you eat", really holds some truth. After eating the same kind of food day in and day out, for years on end, we can permanently take on the energy of the food we have been eating. When food is not good for us, this energy shows up in the form of illness and disease. On the other hand, when we eat well and stay consistent with it, this energy manifests as glowing skin, a healthy smile and most of all, a disease-free body.

WORDS OF WISDOM

What you eat contains chemicals.

What we eat contains chemicals just as drugs do.
Food can be medicine or the wrong medicine can be poison.
For instance, you eat a piece of bacon, however, that pig felt fear
when it was killed in the slaughterhouse. Since emotions come
from hormones (which are triggered in the brain) those chemical
hormones can remain in the meat that you are eating. On an
energetic a level, the negative energy of fear will also deposit into
that meat and into your body. When you continually take this into
our bodies by eating it, imagine what effect it has on us. This is
why eating meat has been commonly connected to emotions of
aggression and anger.

Mood Foods

Improving your mood with the right foods

Feeling lethargic, irritable or tired? Have trouble focusing or sitting still? When this occurs, there is a good chance we are deficient in the minerals our bodies and brain need to function. Too many starchy and cooked foods can make us feel this way. We need to balance our bodies out with live foods including fresh fruits and dark leafy-green vegetables. Out of every meal that we have, 50% of it should consist of fresh vegetables (or fruits in the early morning or late evening). Practicing eating the right foods every day will improve our mood, give us energy, calm our nerves and help us sleep so that we can have a more productive day.

WORDS OF WISDOM

Give your body a break!

We should not eat anything minimum 3-4 hours before we go to sleep. The general rule of thumb is to stop eating at sunset (generally 7/8pm). After this, only drink liquids, or we may eat a piece of fruit. Otherwise, our bodies will be working overtime to digest the food in our stomachs and will not get enough rest. This way we will get the most out of our sleep. Not to mention, once we fall asleep, the food just sits in our gut and begins to ferment in our bodies. When I wake up after eating late, I feel sluggish and heavy. However, when I stick to this rule, even if it is only a few hours of sleep, I feel lighter and more energized!

Deficiencies & Supplements

Ending cravings with proper nutrition

Often, what we tend to crave is not what our bodies need. It is generally a quick fix for something bigger. We are usually missing something important. For example, when I crave bread, pasta or sweets, I am either not getting enough protein or I am deficient in vitamins and minerals. However, when I start my day off with bread or pasta, all I do is crave more bread and pasta. This is simply because those two things are not supplying my body with the necessary nutrients I need, so I start craving something that will give me a quick fix. This is why it is important to start and end our day with fresh fruits, vegetables, and mineral-rich superfoods (like wheatgrass). These items will give our bodies what it needs and curb the cravings. This leads us to supplements. Nutritional supplements make up for what we may not be able to get in our daily meals. In a world where food is losing its nutrients from chemical fertilizers, pesticides, genetic tampering and the long-term abuse of farmland, we have to get our nutrients elsewhere.

Produce in the U.S. and many other parts of the world is not as nutrient-rich as is used to be. We have to supplement by juicing, smoothies and taking supplements.

5 main supplements you may need on plant based diet:
- Vitamin D3
- Vitamin B12
- Biotin (Vitamin H also known as Vitamin B7)
- Omega 3 and 6 (Flaxseed Oil)
- Iodine (Kelp)

EXTRAS: (depending on your body)
- Vitamin C
- Calcium
- Probiotics
- Digestive Enzymes (Papaya Enzymes)
- Multivitamin (made from whole foods)

This handles the crux of our cravings. However, the rest is emotional. Remember this when feeling things out along the journey.

Consult a Naturopathic Doctor or Plant based Nutritionist to find out exactly what you need and the proper dosage. Our bodies are all different and require different things to sustain themselves.

WORDS OF WISDOM

Do not overthink it

You do not have to have a cabinet full of supplements and herbs to be healthy. We have to let food be our medicine. When our bodies are free from blockages resulting from unhealthy foods, it will be able to take in the healing effects of supplements, herbs, spices and foods more effectively.

The Eating Lifestyle Cycle

Understanding the bigger picture

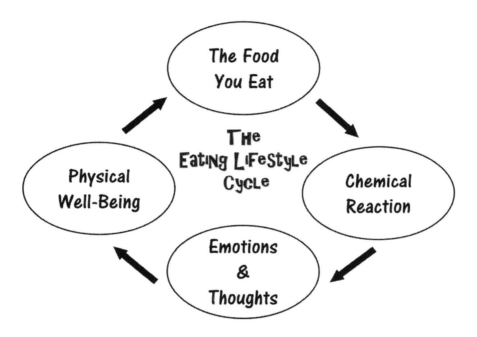

We are what we eat? In a sense, yes! Eating food creates a chemical reaction in our bodies. The chemicals released create a reaction in the brain and manifest as feelings or emotions. Emotions are basically the way our bodies tells us to pay attention to something that may be hurting or helping it. Our emotional state also directly affects our thoughts. Ever had "brain fog"? It may be directly connected to what we eat. These chemicals that make us feel some kind of way also travel through the bloodstream and into the rest of our organs. What we feel in our bodies, then tells us what to eat. This is what I call, the "Eating Lifestyle Cycle." It starts with food and ends with food. This is why, watching our thoughts, what, and how we eat is so important.

The Façade of Losing Weight

Never Count Calories Again!

We tend to focus too much on trying to reach our ideal weight. On every corner we turn, there is a new advertisement about a quick weight loss program or product that will burn off fat in minutes. Though the effects of these things may be great, we need to focus on the core of what is going on in the body as opposed to what lies on the surface. Yes, obesity is an issue in the United States. However, we should not be focused on how we look, but how we feel. Our bodies are the physical manifestations of our thoughts and feelings. When we eat better, we feel better. When we focus on striving to feel our best, our bodies follow suit. In other words, when we feel amazing, we look amazing. There is no need to count calories. When we eat well, our cholesterol and body fat will melt away. So, let us focus on what we can do today to make ourselves feel better. Before we know it, we will look as amazing as we feel.

A Numbers Game

How eating right can save us money

When most of us think about buying healthier food (such as organic ingredients), one of the first complaints we have is about how much more it costs. A regular apple may cost around 50 cents while an organic apple may cost up to $2. After a while, this can add up. However, when we pay the extra amount to eat what makes us feel better, we are actually investing in ourselves. For example, say you spend $50 extra every week buying healthier food. In one month, (since there are usually 4 weeks in a month) that is somewhere around $200 extra we would be spending. There are about 52 weeks in a year so we multiply $50 x 52 weeks and we estimate spending around $2,600 more in one year on eating healthier food. This may seem like a lot, but here are some other numbers to consider before we go all crazy here.

On the flipside of the coin, when we begin to follow a more basic yet healthy eating lifestyle, we end up spending less money. When I started eating more raw foods, I found that I was full more quickly than when I was eating meat and french fries. Honestly, when I was eating heavy meat and starches, I would crave more no matter how full I was. Eating properly means that we get all of the nutrients our bodies need, which curbs our cravings and leaves us feeling satisfied much sooner. In turn, we will be eating less to feel full. Thus, a plate of fresh vegetables and grains costs less than a plate of steak and potatoes.

We usually go the emergency room when we are having an immediate, and usually painful situation that either a doctor cannot fix or that we can simply not wait to go to the doctor for. This applies to something as simple as a really bad stomach ache to severe migraines and stomach pains. The three things I just mentioned are also potential symptoms of more severe, life-altering, diseases such as hernias, tumors or cancer.

The average cost to go to the Emergency Room is about $1,233 a visit. If we were to make two trips to the E.R. in a year, the total would come out to somewhere around $2,466. This is not far off from the estimated $2,600 extra that you would spend to eat better for a year. The biggest difference is that one leaves we feel miserable while the other improves the quality of your life. Are we really willing to sacrifice money for our well-being? Let us consider the idea of feeling amazing. Feeling energized means that we can be more productive. Being more productive means that we can actually make more money. Even though money is not the goal here, the truth is that we make more money when we are healthier than we do when we are not. We cannot be productive when we are sick. So, we have to ask ourselves, *"Is it really money that is keeping us from eating better, or is it our mindset?"*

How much would we be willing to spend to live a longer and happier life? How much is it worth to feel better? How much would we spend to keep from going to the E.R.? It is completely up to us!

WORDS OF WISDOM

Prevention vs. Emergency

Many of us end up in the hospital or the doctor's office thinking, "How did I get here?" I have seen too many people speak about their chronic conditions and terminal illness (such as diabetes and cancer) as if it were bound to happen eventually or were simply something that would happen by chance. This way of thinking is completely false. Do not just let life happen to you. Be the one who chooses what happens in your life. Diseases are preventable. Why wait until we are already sick to make the change?

Location Location Location

Food's connection to our ancestry

Where we are from, where our ancestors are from and where we live all play a role in how your body metabolizes different foods. Why do you think melanated people are more prone to being lactose intolerant and those who are of European descent are more prone to having Celiac Disease? Why is it that people in India and East Africa metabolize bananas better than people in the United States? The answer to these questions is simple. We were created to eat foods that are native to our land and our ancestry. When we ignore this simple fact, our bodies react to let us know that we are not eating properly. Hence, diabetes, gluten-intolerance, Celiac disease, indigestion, chronic ulcers and many other diseases and illnesses pop up as signs that we are not treating our bodies well.

Eating locally and seasonally is one way to prevent this as well as researching our ancestry and learning what they ate. For example, I am half Iranian, and fava beans are a big part of our diet. When I eat beans every now and then, I tend to not have any problems digesting them. However, my friend, who is East African does not do so well eating fava beans or beans in general. Though we both live in the United States, we are predisposed to tolerating certain foods. In short, where we are from and where we live now affects what we should choose to eat.

The Cultural & Social Kick

Eating well without sacrificing your social life

I have found that the hardest part of this process is often breaking the cultural and social stigma. When something is part of our culture and it was the way we were raised, things get difficult; especially if we are still living at home. For example, Dominicans and Brazilians drink coffee. Persians drink black tea. Not to mention, it can get more difficult in a social setting where everyone else is eating or drinking something and we are not. This is where preparation comes into play.

Either we can:

a) Bring our own food/drinks (there have been times where I even bring my own dessert to a restaurant and slip it to the waiter so they can serve it to me with everyone else's).

b) Research a place where everyone can get what they want including us.

c) Change our circles and get around people who are also into eating better (of course we cannot change our family, so we will have to make some adjustments. We can always introduce them to healthier eating habits as well little by little).

The idea that we are less of a __ *(fill in ethnicity here)__* because we do not eat or drink a staple food or beverage is a tough hurdle to get over. However, if you value our health and that of our family, we will overcome it. In reality, we can still honor those cultural traditions, only with a healthy twist. Though it may not be exactly the same, we can still enjoy ourselves in social settings where we may feel awkward. For example, replacing our wine with sparkling cider, or our coffee with a good coffee substitute (hot cocoa or chicory coffee). We can wake up and have our morning cup without sacrificing the ritual.

Traditional food that we eat is not the same today as it was then and in its place of origin. For example, the chicken that may be in our favorite dish today is being fed hormones and antibiotics as opposed to decades ago when they were happily running around in our great grandparent's backyard.

In many cultures what we are traditionally eating today came from throw away foods under impoverished circumstances. Examples of these are animal scraps such as chitterlings (intestines) and pig's feet. Other examples include starchy and filling foods like rice, corn, fufu and bread. These foods have remained as a staple in our diets, however, they are not that healthy for the body. If we can change our poor thinking and poor diet. We will no longer have poor health.

Non-GMO
&
Organic

Why the Hype?

Today, most produce we see in the grocery stores has been genetically modified and sprayed with insecticides and pesticides. The problem with genetically modifying what we eat is that GMO's have not been in existence long enough to be tested on humans. Our bodies do not agree well with genetically modified foods, especially on a long-term basis. Often, our bodies do not completely recognize genetically modified foods as actual food. This means that they take a toll on our digestive and immune systems. Over time, this leads to more chronic, serious and possible life-threatening issues. So, we must ask ourselves this question, "Why would the genetic modification of my food not affect my health?"

Moreover, pesticides and insecticides that are used to kill the bugs that eat away at crops end up in our food. These harmful chemicals that are used to kill living things build up in our bodies over time and become detrimental to our health. These chemicals also eat away at the nutrients in the crops, making them less flavorful and nutritious. So, we think we are getting a considerable amount of nutrients while eating an apple, but that apple may have only 60% of the nutrients it originally had. When reading labels, look for products that are organic and non-GMO (Non Genetically Modified Organisms). Take into account that government standards for who can label their products as organic continue to change. For example, producers can get away with using a slight amount of pesticides on their crops and still call it *organic*. Therefore, continue to do your research on the rules and regulations put on our produce since these tend to change regularly.

Non-GMO: It has not been genetically modified and is, therefore, in its regular state that nature created it. Remember, just because a product is labeled as Non-GMO does not mean that it is *organic*.

Organic: Pesticides and insecticides are not in your food and it is also Non-GMO.
Examine this when shopping at the grocery store food and be sure to buy organic.

If we cannot buy organic produce for any reason, we can use the following recipe until we can:

Stir 1 teaspoon of sea salt and 1 teaspoon of Apple Cider Vinegar in 3-8 cups of warm, purified water. Soak your fruits or vegetables in this solution for 10 minutes. Then rinse and wash well. Though it does not turn your food into organic produce, this will help remove some of the toxins from your food.

There are certain foods that soak up pesticides like sponges. These are especially fruits and vegetables with soft skin. We want to do our best to avoid these unless they are organic. A few of these include

- Cherries
- Strawberries
- Peaches
- Grapes
- Apples
- Nectarines
- Pears
- Lettuce
- Spinach
- Celery
- Sweet Bell Peppers
- Potatoes

Some fruits and vegetables have thick skins (such as avocadoes, mangos, oranges and lemons) which protect the fleshy fruit under these skins from soaking in all of the pesticides. If we cannot buy organic produce for any reason, foods in this category are a bit safer.

40

Inflammatory
&
Mucus Causing
Foods

Combating chronic inflammation

Allergy symptoms such as sneezing, runny nose, coughing and watery eyes is the way our bodies remove particles and harmful bacteria. Mucus is one way our bodies naturally carry harmful bacteria and particles out of the body. The only problem is that, when we eat improperly, the body creates excess mucus as a defensive response. Over time, this excess mucus can lead to many health problems and can even crystalize in the body creating cysts and tumors.

Almost any time we have excess mucus we will find inflammation. They generally occur in the same place (wherever we are experiencing problems). This results in the swelling of any area of the body including the gums, skin, joints and internal organs. Ultimately, contributing to the symptoms of most diseases including crohn's disease, arthritis, eczema and asthma.

Inflammation happens when blood rushes to a certain region of the body and stays there. It is the body's way of giving a certain part of it extra attention so that it can heal. When inflammation is caused by eating improperly it can lead to chronic health conditions. At some point, our bodies do not recognize what we eat as food and attacks it as if it were an invader in the body (the same way it would attack a cold or flu virus). In turn, we begin to feel sick, drained and lethargic. In relation to inflammation in the brain, this can lead to having a lack of concentration and mental disorders. When inflammation takes place in the gut (which it often does when it is food-related), our bodies have trouble absorbing the necessary nutrients from what we eat. This leads to vitamin and mineral deficiencies that negatively affect our overall health and well-being.

Some of the long-term side effects of chronic inflammation include:

- Arthritis
- Irritable Bowel Syndrome
- Crohn's Disease
- Heart Disease
- Cancer
- Asthma
- Sleep Apnea
- Insomnia
- Periodontal Disease (Swelling of the gums)
- Obesity
- Psoriasis
- Eczema
- Osteoporosis (Weak, brittle bones)
- Depression

Below is a short list of inflammatory and mucus-forming foods:

- Dairy and dairy products
- Corn and corn products
- Eggs
- Red Meat
- White Sugar
- Excess Cane Sugar (unrefined)
- Wheat
- Refined Grains (white flour, white rice, etc....)
- Fried foods
- Processed foods (store-bought pastries, pasta, bread, etc....)
- Soy
- Common Cooking Oils (canola, grape seed, cottonseed, safflower, corn and sunflower oils)
- Artificial Additives (food coloring, flavoring and preservatives)
- Alcohol
- Caffeine
- Nuts and nut butters (eat in moderation and separate from other foods)

On another note, we can combat inflammation and excess mucus with these foods:

- Dark leafy green vegetables (kale, spinach, broccoli, etc.)
- Garlic
- Onions
- Ginger
- Turmeric (fresh or dried)
- Radishes (red radish, horseradish, etc.)
- Citrus fruits
- Pineapple (fresh, not canned)
- Berries (in season)
- Peppers (cayenne, jalapeno, etc.)
- Beets
- Coconut Oil
- Flaxseeds
- Chia Seeds

This is simply an abbreviated list and these foods are best when eaten as fresh and unprocessed as possible. The cleaner we eat, the more we will be clear of chronic inflammation and mucus buildup. We will think more clearly, feel more energized throughout the day and be able to fight off disease with ease. Interestingly enough most of these foods are also natural pain relievers. This is because the majority of our pain and discomfort stems from inflammation as a symptom of disease, not the root cause. Once we remove inflammation, pain will cease to exist.

Alkaline vs. Acid-Forming Foods

No longer be prone to disease

When the body is predominately acidic, it is prone to disease. Cancer cells, fungi (such as candida) and other diseases cannot survive in an environment that is alkaline.

Not all foods are alkaline and it would be ridiculous to ask someone to avoid everything that is acidic in nature. However, there should be a balance more on the alkaline side of things. This way, the body can be in a better position to fight off diseases.
When our bodies are acidic, it creates mucus and inflammation. This takes away from our level of energy, causes aging, and can eventually result in cysts, tumors or other long-term, debilitating diseases.

Examples of acidic foods are:
- Meat
- Rice
- Corn
- Wheat
- Oats
- Bread
- Cereal
- Beans (unless sprouted)
- Dairy
- Nuts

- Caffeinated Drinks
- Soy Products
- Sweeteners
- White Sugar
- Table Salt
- White Vinegar

An easy way to remember what is alkaline vs. acid forming is by remembering that **acid-forming foods include most:**
- Grains
- Beans
- Meats
- Dairy Products
- Fish
- Fast Foods
- Fried Foods
- Processed Foods

Alkaline-forming foods include most:
- Fruits
- Vegetables
- Herbs
- Nuts
- Seeds
- Herbal Teas

Try to stay more on the "Alkaline" side as much as possible. This is how we bring the balance. Do we see a trend here? Foods that cause mucus and inflammation are dominantly acidic and the ones that reverse this are alkaline in nature. If we stick to replacing the unhealthy foods with healthier, fresher produce, we will be able to cover all of our bases without overthinking it.

Supplements such as spirulina (a blue-green algae) and wheatgrass are great supplements that can alkalize our bodies on the go. They are available in powdered form and are easy to use when mixed with juice or water.

On the following page is a list of highly alkaline foods. We should do our best to make these at least 80% of what we eat on a daily basis. They will balance any acidity caused by stress, worry, lack of sleep, and eating acid forming foods. Keep in mind that once we expose any of these ingredients to high heat, they lose many of their healing properties and often become acid-forming. Most proteins, when soaked or sprouted maintain the nutritional value. Some must be cooked or sprouted before they can be eaten (such as lentils, quinoa and millet).

ALKALINE FOODS:

VEGETABLES	FRUITS	PROTEINS	OTHER
Artichokes	Avocado	Almonds	Almond Milk
Arugula	Coconut	Amaranth	(raw)
Asparagus	Cucumber	Buckwheat	Avocado Oil
Basil (fresh)	Eggplant	Chia Seeds	Cumin
Beetroot	Grapefruit	Flax Seeds	Flaxseed Oil
Broccoli	Lemon	Lentils	Goats Milk
Brussels Sprouts	Limes	Lima Beans	Olive Oil
Cabbage	Okra	Millet	Sea Moss and
Carrots	Peppers	Mung Beans	Algae
Cauliflower	Pomegranate	Navy Beans	Sprouts (all
Celery	Pumpkin	Peas	kinds)
Chives	Squash	Quinoa	Wheatgrass
Cilantro	Tomatoes	Red Beans	
Collards	Zucchini	Sesame Seeds	
Dandelion		Sunflower	
Greens		Seeds	
Endive			
Garlic			
Green Beans			
Kale			
Kelp			
Leeks			
Lettuce			
Mustard Greens			
Onions			
Parsley			
Radish			
Rhubarb			
Spinach			
Sweet Potatoes			
Swiss Chard			
Thyme (fresh)			
Watercress			

Alkaline Water

What you need to know

Many people choose to drink alkaline water to help balance the acidity in their bodies. Keep in mind that even though this may help, it is not a means to an end. Eating alkaline foods helps give the body energy while removing disease-causing free radicals. Moreover, it is important to know that ionizers (the machines that make alkaline water) do not filter out all of the harmful chemicals in our water. It is best to drink alkaline water from a natural source, such as spring water.

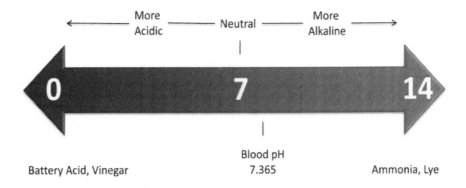

When purchasing alkaline water, we will realize that it has a pH number on it. Alkaline water can be anywhere between 7.5 and 9. Our drinking water should be no higher than a pH of 9 (too alkaline) or lower than 6 (too acidic), otherwise, it can be harmful to our health. Battery acid and vinegar are examples of acids that fall between a pH of 0 and 4. Ammonia and lye are examples of alkaline products that fall between a pH of 11 and 14. The natural pH of our blood is around 7.365, which is almost neutral, but slightly alkaline. We can give our bodies what they need to maintain this level of alkalinity through proper diet and lifestyle.

Our tap water is generally alkaline after adding chlorine to the water to help kill harmful bacteria. However, the chemicals and bacteria remaining in tap water is not the best for our health. Most bottled water (distilled, reverse osmosis, spring, etc.) is slightly acidic. Lemon juice and apple cider vinegar are exceptions when it comes to acid-forming liquids because they actually help alkalize the body once digested. This is why it is good to add a teaspoon of fresh lemon juice or apple cider vinegar to your drinking water to alkalize it. Most artesian bottled water sources are also clean and alkaline in nature.

*Important: Alkaline water boosts the effect of medication and medicinal herbs in the body. To be safe, do not drink alkaline water with medication as well as 30 minutes before or 2 hours after taking anything medicinal. On the other hand, taking vitamin supplements with alkaline water is great since it will increase your absorption rate!

WORDS OF WISDOM

Remedy for indigestion

If we are experiencing indigestion, stir 2 to 5 capfuls of apple cider vinegar in a glass of warm, purified/spring water. This will help balance acid in the stomach.

52

Water Therapy

The dehydration cure

Our bodies are made up of about 60% water. So, it is understandable why getting enough water on a daily basis is critical to our health and well-being. When our bodies get enough water, our internal and external organs can work properly. When we do not get enough water, we become dehydrated. Dehydration causes more issues than we give credit to.

When your body is trying to remove toxins, it needs water to make that happen. These toxins will then flush our through your urine and fecal matter. Without enough water, our bodies are unable to remove these toxins and this eventually results in a buildup of toxicity within the body. This buildup is one of the main culprits in causing disease.

It varies by weight and how much you sweat every day, but the general rule of thumb is to drink eight 8-ounce glasses (equivalent to four 16-ounce glasses) of water a day. Or, two-thirds of your body weight in ounces. One great way to keep track of your water intake is to buy a ½ gallon jug or 2 liter bottle, fill it with water, and make sure to finish it by the end of the day. We can carry the jug around with us or we can fill up a water bottle (or two) with the water that was in the jug when we know we are about to go out. This way, the jug is not as weighty. When we get back home, finish the jug. If we end up drinking more water then was in our jug, then great! This is a way to help us reach our *minimum* water intake.

When we first wake up, before we brushing our teeth, eating, or drinking anything, it is important that we drink four to six 8-ounce glasses of warm lemon (or lime) water to open up our digestive system. Start off by heating up distilled, reverse osmosis, spring or alkaline water in a tea kettle until it begins to steam. Squeeze half a lemon or lime into the bottom of your glass. Then fill up half of your glass with the hot water and top it off with your room temperature purified water. Drink 6 of these glasses within a 15-minute period (back-to-back if possible). Alternatively, if we cannot drink 6 glasses first thing in the morning, then we can start off with two and working our way up over the next few weeks.

The lemon (or lime) juice balances the acidity within the body as it enters the stomach. Apple Cider Vinegar is also an option, but I have found it to be a bit more abrasive than the lemon. Wait at least 30 min after doing this before you eat anything. If you do not wait, you may have trouble digesting your food.

When it comes to water, spring water is the best option. Nature has made it so that spring water has the perfect pH level and all the minerals your body needs to be completely rehydrated. Keep in mind that many big companies are filling their bottles with fluoridated water and calling it spring water. This is why it is important to be aware and do your research. If it is possible, support small business and buy local. This will circumvent this problem.

Notice how I did not include tap water in the instructions. The negative long-term effects of drinking tap water are discussed in this book. However, if you are unable to get access to any form of purified water, boil your tap water for 2-5 minutes and let it stand (preferably in sunlight) for one hour. Then, boil it again immediately before using it. Doing this while adding fresh-squeezed lemon juice will help balance and cleanse your water until you can get access to something that is cleaner.

This is a great way to slowly wake up the body while rehydrating, alkalizing and purifying the internal organs. Water therapy has helped me with constipation or infrequent bowel movements, grogginess, brain fog, allergies, eczema, asthma, flu symptoms and a multitude of other symptoms that I would possibly be experiencing throughout the day.

*Do not use a microwave

**Make sure to do this at least an hour before you have to leave the house, practicing this will send you to the bathroom a couple of times.

WORDS OF WISDOM

Drink water at room temperature.

When we constantly drink cold water, our bodies have to work harder to maintain its internal temperature. This puts the body under undue stress. To keep our immune systems strong and add a few years to our lives, keep the container of purified water out of the refrigerator and do not add ice.

WORDS OF WISDOM:

Drinking while eating

Try not to drink beverages within an hour before or after you eat. This includes drinking while we are eating. We all like the idea of "washing it down" with an ice-cold beverage, however, this slows down the digestive process and this takes a toll on the body. We will also end up with less energy. Drinking cold beverages also stresses the body. Our bodies are naturally warm and introducing something cold into the system puts it in shock. This will speed up the aging process. Drinking warm or hot liquids when it is hot out may seem counter-intuitive. Conversely, doing this regulates our internal body temperature, making us sweat and consequently, feeling cooler. This is why we may often see people from Eastern cultures, who come from warmer areas that are closer to the equator, drink hot teas year-round.

Edible Foods

More is not always better

When our protein bar has over 15 ingredients in it, we may have to question if it is really good for us. Just because things like these have healthy ingredients does not mean it is a good thing. Our bodies are only meant to digest a few things at a time. Too many additives can diminish the natural healing properties of plants. So, the fewer ingredients on the ingredient label, the easier it is on the body.

Think about it like this. "Bar X" has an ingredient list containing 15 organic ingredients. These include soy protein, rice flour, rolled oats, cane sugar, chocolate liquor, cocoa butter, soy lecithin, vanilla, tapioca syrup, agave syrup, arabic gum, almonds, tapioca, flaxseed and natural flavors. Now, imagine all of these ingredients separately stacked on a plate in front of you. Could you imagine eating all of these in one sitting without getting a stomach ache? Most of us cannot. The amazing thing is that this is one of the simpler ingredient lists. The majority of "healthy" products out there contain 30 ingredients or more.

58

Food Combining

The indigestion cure

Practicing proper food combining can help with digestive issues such as indigestion, gas, bloating and constipation. It can also alleviate other symptoms as a result of long-term indigestion such as ulcers, depression and trouble breathing.

When I began to practice proper food combining, I realized that I felt lighter and more energized after meals. I also had a much easier time eliminating waste on a regular basis. The fun part about food combining is that it pushes me to be more creative when planning meals, since many conventional recipes are not in line with proper food combining.

WORDS OF WISDOM

Simplicity is key!

Many of us have digestive issues because we put too many things together at the same time. This puts extra stress on the body. Not to mention, the healing properties in the foods we eat are diminished when we add too many unnecessary ingredients. The most common place I see this in when we make smoothies. Just because every ingredient in the blender is healthy does not mean it is healthy together. The wrong combination of fruits, vegetables and proteins can be a recipe for disaster. This is why it is important to know how to combine foods properly.

Proteins
Proteins should be eaten alone and they should not be paired with other proteins. For example, lentils can be eaten alone as a soup; however, lentils and beans together would be difficult to digest. One of my favorite meals is lentil soup with a spinach salad. The spinach is fine since it is a leafy green vegetable and goes with almost everything.

After eating proteins, wait about 3-4 hours for them to digest before introducing starches, fruits or other proteins into your diet.

Starches
When eating starches, half of the digestion process takes place in the mouth. As we chew our food, the enzymes in our saliva begin to break down these starches in ways that our stomachs cannot. This is why it is important to take our time and chew. Otherwise, these grains simply pass through our system, undigested. This can lead to deficiencies and constipation.

Why do we get gassy after eating pastries such as cookies, cakes and pies? When we eat sugar, it starts a reaction in our salivary glands telling our bodies not to produce the enzymes that help break down starches. In other words, sugar tricks our bodies into thinking the starches that we are eating (from the flours in our pastries) are not there. So, the chemicals that break down these starches are not excreted. This is why sugars and starches should not be eaten together. Instead of adding sugar to our oatmeal in the morning, a savory oatmeal recipe would be a great alternative.

The problem with beans is that they are equally starch and protein within themselves. So, the body has trouble completely digesting beans for this reason alone. However, soaking, sprouting or fermenting beans helps. Though this does not completely eliminate this ordeal.

After eating starches, wait at least 2-3 hours for them to digest before introducing proteins, fruits, or sugars into your diet.

Vegetables

Dark leafy green vegetables such as spinach, kale, collards, mustard greens and dandelion greens can be combined with anything and will actually assist in digestion. Herbs and roots such as basil, peppermint and ginger can also be combined with anything to assist in digestion. Vegetables are great when paired with starches such as eating broccoli with brown rice. They also pair well with proteins, such as combining cauliflower with millet.

Fruits

Out of all foods, fruit digests the fastest and should always be eaten on an empty stomach *at least 30 minutes to an hour before eating anything else.* This is why fruit is great to eat in the morning since it is easy on the body while we are waking up.

At family reunions, we would always eat watermelon to close out a big meal. I would always wonder why I would feel so tired and bloated afterwards. I simply could not understand why eating something so light would make me feel so heavy. The reason is that melons, out of all fruits, digest the fastest and should only be eaten on an empty stomach (generally first thing in the morning). When we eat a melon after a meal full of starches and proteins, the stomach is busy breaking down the proteins of the other foods that take much longer to digest. So, this fruit simply sits on top of everything else, adding extra weight and eventually fermenting, creating gas in the stomach and gut. Examples of melons include watermelon, honeydew and cantaloupe. Remember that melons should not be combined with other foods, including other fruits.

Remember that there are different categories for fruits, and it is helpful to eat these separately as well. These include:

SWEET FRUITS:
Bananas, Dates, Figs, Muscat Grapes, Papaya, Persimmons
SUB-ACID FRUITS:
Apples, Blackberries, Blueberries, Cherries, Grapes (red, black and green varieties), Mangoes, Nectarines, Peaches, Pears, Plums, Raspberries
ACID FRUITS: (includes most citrus fruits)
Cranberries, Grapefruits, Kiwi, Lemons, Limes, Oranges, Pineapples, Pomegranates, Strawberries, Tangerines, Tomatoes
HIGH FAT FRUITS:
Avocado, Olives, Coconut
NON-SWEET FRUITS (FRUIT-VEGETABLES)
Bell Peppers, Cucumbers, Tomatoes, Squash, Eggplants, Okra, Zucchini, Plantains

Did you know that there is a category of vegetables that are actually fruits? These fruit-vegetables should be eaten together and not combined with other sweet and citrus fruits. Examples of these are cucumbers, okra, tomatoes, zucchinis, peppers and plantains. Be aware that, combining fruit-vegetables with proteins, starches or other starchy vegetables can cause gas and indigestion.

Do not mix fruits with vegetables, especially starchy vegetables since they require different acidic environments in the stomach to fully digest. Salads with fruit in them are very popular. However, I always wondered why I would feel gassy after eating a big salad with spinach, avocadoes, cucumbers, raspberries and mandarin orange slices in it. It was simply because the fruits and vegetables did not blend well in my stomach.

After eating fruits, wait about 30 minutes to an hour for them to digest before introducing proteins, starches or vegetables into your diet. The same stand for vegetables.

Remember that *this is a process.* There is no need to feel overwhelmed. We can even take it and apply what we can piece by piece. For example, now that we know that proteins should not be combined with other proteins, we can start by making our meals simpler with only one protein instead of two. As we continue to apply this information, it will get easier to remember what goes together and what does not. We will begin to become a whizzes at creating new recipes that work for US. We will be on our way to feeling lighter and more energized after every meal.

This process is about awareness, not obsession. Awareness of how we eat and how it affects our bodies is the first step to optimal health. When we obsess over these things, we can make ourselves sick. Then we experience a placebo-like effect where we are so fixated on how bad something is for us that we feel ill simply thinking about it. The key here is mind over matter. When we envision something, the body will follow. So, instead we must affirm in our beings that we are well, and that we are healing through consistent practice.

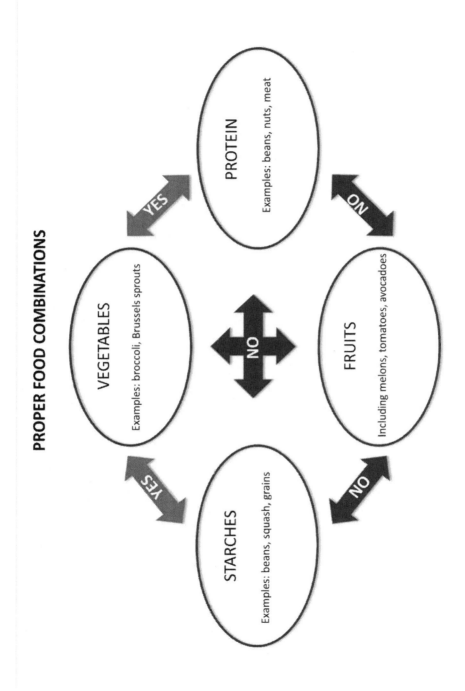

Eating In Season

Getting the most out of your food

Why eat in season? The real question should be, why not?
The land that we are standing on naturally creates certain fruits and vegetables that help our bodies cope with the changes of each season. For example, in the United States, brussels sprouts are in season in the winter. They are high in Vitamin C, which help fight off disease during the cold months, and minerals such as magnesium, which regulates body temperature.

Also, eating in season means our food is fresh. Fruits and vegetables are in their ripest state when they are in season. Eating fresh, ripe, local produce means that we are getting the most nutrients (and flavor) out of our food.

*If we live outside the United States, make sure to look up seasonal foods of that country since some of the foods on this chart may differ.

*This is a general list of foods in their peak season by month in the United States. Look up seasonal foods in each region since the regions may differ in harvesting. For example, crops in southern California tend to be in their peak season much longer than those in North Carolina. Look up a "seasonal food guide" online for each state.

If we are going to eat in season, read the labels when shopping to make sure the produce is locally grown or at least grown in our home countries. The point of eating seasonally is to get the most out of fresh, local produce. When produce is imported, it is usually because it is not native to our land or it is simply out of season in our area.

Look at the current month to see what fruits and vegetables are in their peak season in the United States. If we do not recognize some of these, look them up. Each of these fruits and vegetables have their own set of health benefits. This is a chance to try something new and add a little variety to our diet. We may even find a new favorite food!
Be mindful that dried legumes including beans, grains and seeds are in season year-round.

Obviously, this is an abbreviated list and we should continue to look into other fruits and vegetables that are not on the list to see when they are in season as well. Use the following guide when shopping and planning meals.

JANUARY

Vegetables	Fruits
broccoli	grapefruit
broccolini	kiwi
brussels sprouts	oranges
butternut squash	pomegranate
celery	tangerines
collards	
fennel	
kale	
leeks	
lamb's lettuce	
potatoes	
pumpkin	
rutabaga	
sweet potatoes	
sunchoke	
turnips	

FEBRUARY

Vegetables	Fruits
broccoli	grapefruit
broccolini	kiwi
brussels sprouts	oranges
butternut squash	tangerines
celery	
collards	
fennel	
kale	
leeks	
lamb's lettuce	
potatoes	
rutabaga	
sunchoke	
turnips	

MARCH

Vegetables	Fruits
broccoli	blood oranges
broccolini	grapefruit
celery	kiwi
fennel	oranges
kale	pineapple
leeks	
lamb's lettuce	
potatoes	
rutabaga	
sunchoke	
turnips	

APRIL

Vegetables	Fruits
artichoke	blood oranges
asparagus	grapefruit
avocado	kiwi
broccoli	pineapple
fava beans	
kale	
peas	
radishes	
rhubarb	
turnips	

MAY

Vegetables	Fruits
artichoke	apricots
asparagus	grapefruit
avocado	kiwi
broccoli	lemons
corn	limes
cucumber	pineapple
fava beans	strawberries
peas, radishes	
rhubarb	
spinach	
zucchini	

JUNE

Vegetables	Fruits
arugula	apricots
asparagus	blueberries
bell peppers	cherries
carrots	grapefruit
corn	lemons
cucumber	limes
peas	melon
radishes	passion fruit
rhubarb	pineapple
spinach	plums
zucchini	strawberries

JULY

Vegetables	Fruits
arugula	apricots
beets	blackberries
beet greens	blueberries
bell peppers	cherries
carrots	lemons
corn	limes
cucumber	melon
eggplant	mulberries
garlic	nectarines
peas	passion fruit
radishes	peaches
rhubarb	plums
zucchini	strawberries
	tomatoes

AUGUST

Vegetables	Fruits
artichoke	apricots
arugula	blackberries
beets	blueberries
beet greens	figs
bell peppers	lemons
carrots	limes
cauliflower	melon
corn	mulberries
eggplant	nectarines
garlic	peaches
radishes	plums
rhubarb	tomatoes
sweet potatoes	
zucchini	

SEPTEMBER

Vegetables	Fruits
artichoke	almonds
beets	apples
beet greens	chestnuts
bell peppers	cranberries
carrots	limes
cauliflower	melon
corn	pears
eggplant	plums
garlic	pomegranate
potatoes	raspberries
radishes	tomatoes
sweet potatoes	
wild mushrooms	

OCTOBER

Vegetables	Fruits
artichoke	almonds
bell peppers	apples
beets	chestnuts
beet greens	cranberries
broccolini	limes
brussels sprouts	pears
butternut squash	plums
cauliflower	pomegranate
carrots	tomatoes
celery	
chard	
fennel	
garlic	
leeks	
parsnip	
potatoes	
pumpkin	
radishes	
spinach	
sweet potatoes	
wild mushrooms	

NOVEMBER

Vegetables	Fruits
bell peppers	almonds
broccoli	apples
broccolini	chestnuts
brussels sprouts	cranberries
butternut squash	kiwi
cauliflower	pears
celery	persimmon
chard	pomegranate
collards	tangerines
fennel	
garlic	
leeks	
parsnip	
potatoes	
pumpkin	
rutabaga	
spinach	
sweet potatoes	
sunchoke	
turnips	
wild mushrooms	

DECEMBER

Vegetables	Fruits
broccoli	cranberries
broccolini	kiwi
brussels sprouts	oranges
butternut squash	persimmon
cauliflower	pomegranate
celery	tangerines
collards	
fennel	
leeks	
lamb's lettuce	
potatoes	
pumpkin	
rutabaga	
sweet potatoes	
sunchoke	
turnips	

The following pages contain seasonal food charts for quick reference:

SEASONAL FRUITS

JAN	FEB	MAR	APR	MAY	JUN	JULY	AUG	SEPT	OCT	NOV	DEC
Grapefruit	Grapefruit	Blood Oranges	Blood Oranges	Apricots	Apricots	Apricots	Apricots	Almonds	Almonds	Almonds	Cranberries
Kiwi	Kiwi	Grapefruit	Grapefruit	Grapefruit	Blueberries	Blackberries	Blueberries	Apples	Apples	Apples	Kiwi
Oranges	Oranges	Kiwi	Kiwi	Kiwi	Cherries	Blueberries	Blackberries	Chestnuts	Chestnuts	Chestnuts	Oranges
Pomegranate	tangerines	Oranges	Pineapple	Lemons	Grapefruit	Cherries	Figs	Cranberries	Cranberries	Cranberries	Persimmon
Tangerines		Pineapple		Limes	Lemons	Lemons	Lemons	Limes	Limes	Kiwi	Pomegranate
				Pineapple	Limes	Limes	Limes	Melons	Pears	Pears	Tangerines
				Strawberries	Melons	Melons	Melons	Plums	Plums	Persimmon	
					Passionfruit	Mulberries	Mulberries	Pears	Pomegranate	Pomegranate	
					Pineapple	Nectarines	Nectarines	Pomegranate	Tomatoes	Tangerines	
					Plums	Passion Fruit	Peaches	Raspberries			
					Strawberries	Peaches	Plums	Tomatoes			
						Plums	Tomatoes				
						Strawberries					
						Tomatoes					

SEASONAL VEGETABLES

JAN	FEB	MAR	APR	MAY	JUN	JULY	AUG	SEPT	OCT	NOV	DEC
Broccoli	Broccoli	Broccoli	Artichoke	Artichoke	Arugula	Arugula	Artichoke	Artichoke	Artichoke	Bell Peppers	Broccoli
Broccolini	Broccolini	Broccolini	Asparagus	Asparagus	Asparagus	Beets	Arugula	Beets	Beets	Broccoli	Broccolini
Brussels Sprouts	Brussels Sprouts	Celery	Avocado	Avocado	Bell Peppers	Bell Peppers	Beets	Bell Peppers	Bell Peppers	Broccolini	Brussels Sprouts
Butternut Squash	Butternut Squash	Fennel	Broccoli	Broccoli	Carrots	Carrots	Bell Peppers	Carrots	Broccolini	Brussels Sprouts	Butternut Squash
Celery	Celery	Kale	Fava Beans	Corn	Corn	Corn	Carrots	Cauliflower	Brussels Sprouts	Butternut Squash	Cauliflower
Collards	Collards	Leeks	Kale	Cucumber	Cucumber	Cucumber	Cauliflower	Corn	Butternut Squash	Cauliflower	Celery
Fennel	Fennel	Potatoes	Peas	Peas	Peas	Eggplant	Corn	Eggplant	Cauliflower	Celery	Collards
Kale	Kale	Rutabaga	Radishes	Radishes	Radishes	Garlic	Eggplant	Garlic	Carrots	Chard	Fennel
Leeks	Leeks	Salsify	Rhubarb	Rhubarb	Rhubarb	Peas	Garlic	Potatoes	Celery	Collards	Leeks
Potatoes	Potatoes	Sunchoke	Turnips	Spinach	Spinach	Radishes	Radishes	Radishes	Chard	Fennel	Potatoes
Pumpkin	Rutabaga	Turnips		Zucchini	Zucchini	Rhubarb	Rhubarb	Sweet Potatoes	Fennel	Garlic	Pumpkin
Rutabaga	Salsify					Zucchini	Sweet Potatoes	Wild Mushrooms	Garlic	Leeks	Rutabaga
Salsify	Sunchoke						Zucchini		Leeks	Parsnips	Salsify
Sweet Potatoes	Turnips								Parsnips	Potatoes	Sweet Potatoes
Sunchoke									Potatoes	Pumpkin	Sunchoke
Turnips									Pumpkin	Rutabaga	Turnips
									Radishes	Salsify	
									Spinach	Spinach	
									Sweet Potatoes	Sweet Potatoes	
									Wild Mushrooms	Sunchoke	
										Turnips	
										Mushrooms	

WORDS OF WISDOM

50% live foods

Always make sure that your plate includes at least 50% raw fruits or vegetables. The nutrients in the raw foods will have you feeling healthier and you will have less of a tendency to overeat. Once you get used to eating 50% raw, trying going to 60% and then 70%. You can never have too much live food.

Know Your Body

Understanding the digestive process

Since we will be talking about eating, it is important to know about our organs and how they digest food. We will start from the top of the body and go all the way to the bottom.

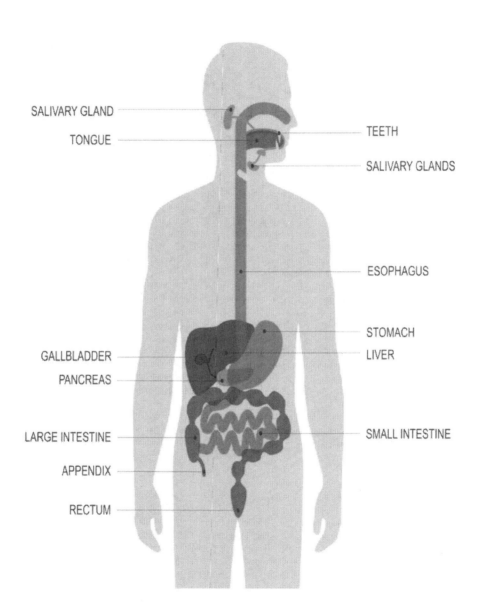

- **Mouth** – The mouth is a big part of digestion that most of us take for granted. When we chew our food, we are breaking it down so that it is easier on our stomachs. Your saliva begins to break down the food even further (with an enzyme called amylase that breaks down the starches).
- **Stomach** – Your stomach acids and enzymes break down the food even further
- **Small Intestine** – The liquid-like food gets broken down even more with enzymes in the small intestine and the fats get dissolved here as well. Food that is broken down enough is absorbed as nutrients into the body.
- **Pancreas** – Creates insulin, which regulates your blood sugar. The pancreas also creates the enzymes for the small intestine, which break down your food.
- **Liver** - The liver processes the nutrients absorbed by the small intestine. It also detoxifies harmful substances that are in the blood (such as bacteria).
- **Large Intestine (aka the Colon)** – The remainder of the food that could not be dissolved into the small intestine is broken down by all of the bacteria in the large intestine. The large intestine is full of healthy bacteria that break down what your stomach and small intestine could not. Whatever can be broken down and used as nutrients for the body is dissolved into the bloodstream and the remainder is pushed further down as solid, fecal matter.
- **Kidneys** – The kidneys constantly clean the blood. They also filter out toxic waste and extra water.
- **Bladder** – The liquid waste from our kidneys is then stored in our bladder in the form of urine.

When we practice a healthy eating lifestyle, all of these organs remain in good health and continue to work at their highest capacity. However, when we do not manage how we eat, these organs begin to break down. This is how we end up with issues such as ulcers, kidney disease and colon cancer. Now that we know the main organs involved in digestion, we can greater understand the impact of how we eat on our health and well-being.

WORDS OF WISDOM

Walking after meals

When possible, take a 15-30 minute walk after each big meal. This will improve digestion by letting gravity do the work and allowing you to feel lighter throughout the day.

Disease Explained

The true definition of disease

Let us break down the word *disease* for a second:

"*Ease*" is a state of physical comfort, tranquility and peace of mind. It is the undisturbed state of the body. When we add the letters "*dis-*" to the beginning of a word (this is called a "prefix" for all you English geeks), it reverses the meaning of the word. So, "*Dis-Ease*" is the opposite of *ease*. We are no longer "*at ease.*" Instead, we are experiencing discomfort, agitation, and chaos. The natural flow in our bodies is disrupted.

Our bodies speak to us every day. When we are healthy and balanced, everything is in working order. When our bodies have a reaction, or we feel pain or discomfort, it is the way the body says, "Hey! Help me out here!" Depending on the type of reaction, including how, when and where it happens, we can tell what is going on inside of us. In most cases, we get early signs for much bigger, life-changing diseases. A good example would be chronic indigestion or a twinge in the stomach, even when we are not eating. The body is communicating to us, "Hey! I do not like what you are doing to my stomach!" If we pay attention to these "tiny" shifts in our bodies, we can address them and possibly prevent something worse from happening. It could be as simple as removing one thing from your diet. However, if we ignore it and continue with our everyday lives (like most of us do), it can progress into something worse, such as Stomach or Colon Cancer.

Begin to pay attention to the little things your body is telling you. Using your journal, take a moment to make a list of all of the aches, pains or other forms of discomfort you are experiencing. You will most likely have to come back and add to this list a couple times. Most of us normalize our pain so that we can focus on getting through the day. This list will help you tackle your forms of dis-ease head on so that you can truly heal. Throughout your healing journey, check off the things you no longer feel. This will show you how far you have really come!

Common Food-Related Diseases, Illnesses and Disorders:

Alzheimer's Disease Dementia (memory loss) Autism Bipolar Disorder ADD and ADHD Addiction (alcohol, tobacco, etc.) Anxiety Depression Low Energy	Gastrointestinal Problems (heartburn, IBS, ulcers etc.) Acid Reflux Hiatal Hernia Crohn's Disease Celiac Disease
Eating Disorders Obesity Diabetes	Hypertension (high blood pressure) Hypotension (low blood pressure) Heart Disease (heart attack, stroke)
Cancer (all forms) Tumors Cystic Fibrosis Uterine Fibroids	Asthma COPD (emphysema, chronic bronchitis) Sleep Apnea Insomnia
Multiple Sclerosis ALS (Lou Gehrig's Disease) Lupus Fibromyalgia	Weakened Vision Astigmatism Glaucoma Cataracts
Dermatitis (Eczema, Psoriasis) Acne Accelerated Aging (wrinkles, graying hairs, etc.) Hair loss	Constipation Hemorrhoids Intestinal Parasites and Worms
Weak Immune System Flu and Cold Ear infections Sore Throat Headaches and Migraines	Infertility Impotence (erectile dysfunction) Incontinence (bladder)
Bacterial Infections (septicemia, etc.) Fungal Infections (athlete's foot, etc.) Candidiasis Oral Health (bleeding gums, sores, cavities, etc.) Unpleasant Body Odor	Arthritis (tendonitis, carpal tunnel, gout swelling in joints, etc.) Pain and Inflammation in Joints Osteoporosis (fragile bones) Back, shoulder and neck pain

90

PART II

Culinary Bondage

What foods are keeping us down + their healthy alternatives

The reality is that *all* diseases are food related. Since what we eat can break down or build up the body. However, the diseases listed on the previous page are the most prominent. The most common and most accessible foods out there are usually the ones that keep us down. The foods that are listed below have fundamental ingredients in them, which keep us in a pattern of disease. The only way to break free from these things is to know better alternatives.

- **Potato Chips** - fried foods, white potatoes, corn, soy, canola oil, table salt, dairy, yeast, artificial flavors, artificial food coloring, artificial preservatives
- **Cookies, Pies and Cakes** - wheat, corn, soy, white potatoes, dairy, eggs, artificial preservatives, food coloring, artificial flavors
- **Cheesy Foods** - dairy, pork products
- **Chocolate** - dairy, sugar, artificial sweetener, soy, artificial preservatives
- **Ice Cream** - dairy, soy, sugar, artificial food color, artificial preservatives
- **Bread** - wheat, corn, soy, white potatoes, dairy, eggs, artificial preservatives, food coloring, artificial flavors
- **Pizza** - wheat, dairy and red meat (often)
- **Cheeseburgers, Hot dogs and Hamburgers** - Wheat, dairy, corn, eggs, soy, red meat
- **Bacon** - red meat
- **Fried Chicken** - white meat, eggs, dairy, corn, wheat, soy, artificial preservatives
- **Breakfast Cereal** - wheat, corn, soy, dairy, artificial flavors, colors and preservatives, excess sugar
- **Steak** - red meat
- **Muffins and Cupcakes** - dairy, eggs, corn, soy, wheat, artificial preservatives, food coloring, artificial flavors, excess sugar and salt
- **Pasta** - wheat, corn, eggs
- **Doughnuts** - dairy, eggs, wheat, excess sugar and salt
- **French Fries** - white potatoes, fried food, eggs, wheat, soy, artificial food coloring, artificial preservatives

- **Candy and Bubble Gum** - sugar, corn, artificial food coloring, artificial preservatives, artificial flavor

Not everything that grows from the earth is for human consumption. For example, certain grains, nuts and seeds were made to be consumed by other animals, not us. **The following pages describe ingredients that keep us in bondage along with their healthy alternatives.**

Corn

The majority of corn we eat today is GMO. Even the labels that say "non GMO" are GMO to a certain extent. In the mid 1990's, mass produced corn was genetically modified to naturally kill the corn worm in order to increase production. So, we should ask ourselves, if it has been changed to kill something, what is it doing inside of our bodies? Of course, if we are going to eat corn, we can do our best to get the "non GMO" version, because it is the healthier alternative.
Sadly, most of the products out there with any form of corn in them (cornstarch, corn syrup, etc.) are GMO.
Rule of thumb- the more processed it is, the worse it is for the body (i.e.: processed cornstarch vs. corn on the cob).

Common corn products (you see on an ingredient label):
- Caramel Color
- Vegetable Cellulose
- Cornmeal
- Cornstarch
- Modified Food Starch
- Corn Syrup
- High Fructose Corn Syrup
- Maltodextrin
- Maltose
- Dextrose
- HVP (Hydrolyzed Vegetable Protein)
- MSG
- Sorbitol
- Xylitol
- Distilled White Vinegar

Eating corn increases chances of diseases such as:

- Infertility
- Cysts and Tumors
- Kidney Failure
- Weak Liver
- Asthma
- Sinus Problems
- Dizziness
- Diabetes
- Headaches
- Indigestion
- Obesity
- Lethargy
- Eczema (rashes on skin)

Wheat

For thousands of years, wheat has been tampered with to increase production and this has had some serious effects on how our bodies take it in. Since the 1960's, the majority of wheat we consume today is a hybridized form of wheat called "dwarf wheat" which has a significantly higher level of gluten in it and lower nutritional value. This is where we come upon the "gluten-free" craze as more and more people are becoming gluten-intolerant or diagnosed with Celiac Disease. This is just a hunch, but I believe that this can be attributed to our bodies "overdosing" on gluten over the past few decades to the point where it forms an intolerance.

Not only do we consume a lot of wheat, but we consume a tremendous amount of wheat with excess amounts of gluten. Gluten and something called WGA (Wheat Germ Agglutinin) which is a chemical within wheat itself, is the key culprit in causing inflammation in the body. For example, wheat gluten is the main ingredient in glue and wallpaper paste and can simply be made by mixing wheat flour with water. Imagine what it is doing inside of our bodies.

Additionally, we no longer allow our grains to ferment and break down the way our ancestors used to. Instead, we eat grains, such as wheat, in an indigestible form which strains our digestive system and eventually leads to disease.

Wheat also triggers the release of dopamine in the body. Dopamine is a feel-good neurotransmitter created by the brain. It makes us feel motivated and happy. This is a great example of how food is medicine. The core issue here is that most of us have overdosed on wheat. This has created certain problems over the course of generations.

To relieve joint pain, we can take wheat out of our diets. Many people take glucosamine tablets to help with their joint pain. Our bodies naturally create glucosamine, however, wheat has a chemical in it that inhibits the ability of the body to process glucosamine in the joints. So, removing wheat from our diets may be one step in the right direction to letting our bodies do what it was created to do and relieving joint pain.

What about Spelt, Kamut and other types of wheat that are not as commonly used? This is a touchy subject because the commercial food industry is using more and more of these products. In turn, mass production leads to tampering with the product in order to produce more. Also, once we have lived a life consuming too much gluten, our bodies cannot tolerate the slightest amount of it. We must give our bodies a break and cleanse it from our system.

List Common wheat products (you see on an ingredient label):
- All-Purpose flour
- White Flour
- Most Bread
- Couscous
- Einkorn
- Farro
- Farina
- Durum
- Einkorn
- Kamut
- Gluten (aka. vital wheat gluten)
- Malt (or malt extract)
- Matzo
- Noodles and Pasta
- Seitan
- Semolina
- Spelt
- Tabbouleh
- Triticale (or Triticum)

Eating wheat increases chances of diseases such as:

- Celiac Disease
- Inflammation
- Malnutrition
- Asthma
- Eczema
- Diabetes
- Heart Disease
- Stroke
- Alzheimer's disease
- Arthritis
- Depression
- Cancer
- Infertility
- Liver Disease
- Weak Immune System
- Constipation
- ADHD

100

Pasta

Most pasta is made from wheat and eggs. Try replacing wheat pasta with rice noodles. Most grocery stores today sell rice noodles. Asian grocery stores and health food stores will usually have the greatest variety of wheat free noodles available. There are other pasta alternative such gluten free pastas that are made brown rice, millet, quinoa.

Recognize that, if we do eat rice, we must eat it in moderation. Too much rice can lead to digestive issues such as constipation. It is also high in carbs, which turn into sugar in the body. This will only make us tired and wanting to eat more. We should always listen to our bodies. We will know what is best for it. Be sure to look out for the brands that do not use corn in their production.

Here is a list of brands that sell gluten free, healthy pasta alternatives:

- Annie's
- Ancient Harvest
- Bionaturae
- Daiya
- DeBoles
- Field Day Organic
- Hodgson Mill
- Tinkyada
- Trader Joe's

102

Soy

When most people think of "vegan" or "vegetarian" food, they think of soy products such as tofu, tempeh and seitan. Soy burgers and hot dogs are used as "transitional meat" in order to make it easier for people who are working towards removing meat from their diets. However, eating soy in excess can cause serious chronic diseases. I knew soy was not good for me once I had fasted from soy products for 6 months. Just after eating a piece of tofu, I would experience tension and discomfort in my spine. One of the reasons I was having a reaction is because soy products contain histamine. Histamine in foods can cause severe allergic reactions including inflammation inside the body and on the skin.

Unless we are not eating meat for ethical reasons, we are better off eating high-quality meat here and there. Even though it is the "lesser of two evils", the negative effects of soy on the body outweigh the negative effects of a properly cooked, high-quality piece of farm-raised chicken.

List Common Soy products (you see on an ingredient label):

- Soybeans
- Edamame
- Soy Protein
- Soy Milk
- Soy Oil
- Lecithin
- Hydrolyzed Vegetable Protein (HVP)
- Miso
- Tempeh
- Teriyaki
- Tamari

- Textured Vegetable Protein (TVP)
- Tofu
- Bean Curd

Eating Soy increases chances of diseases such as:
- Cancer
- Brain Damage
- Infant Abnormalities
- Thyroid Disorders
- Kidney Stones
- Weak Immune System
- Severe Food Allergies / Hay Fever
- Impaired Fertility
- Cystic Fibrosis
- Kidney Failure
- Asthma
- Diabetes

Freedom Factor!
For a healthier option, try eating soy and wheat free veggie burgers. Many companies are beginning to use the pea protein in place of soy and wheat ingredients in their meat substitutes. They have the texture of meat, soy and wheat gluten without the negative health effects. Visit the vegetarian section of the freezer at the grocery store to find some of these tasty alternatives.

Red Meat

Including Pork, Beef and Lamb

Sure, red meat is rich in B vitamins and iron, however, a diet that is dominant in red meat can lead to a number of diseases. It can take up to 72 hours for red meat to leave our digestive tract, leaving us feeling quite heavy and taxed. The biggest culprit I would say is not the red meat itself, but how it is prepared. Most red meat involves cuts that are high in cholesterol-raising fats which are then grilled or fried in oil. After years of eating like this, it is no wonder why people with this diet have cardiovascular issues. These days, pork is in everything. Ranging from breakfast foods to chocolate. Our nation is addicted to the pig. However, pork is one of the main factors when it comes to food-related disease. Pigs are bottom-feeders, eating almost anything in their path. Pigs will even eat other dead animal parts when they are hungry enough. Pork, along with other forms of meat are pumped with antibiotics and growth hormones. Due to their imbalanced diets, their meat is more prone to being infected with worms and other harmful bacteria, which if not stored and cooked correctly can replicate itself in your gut.

List of Common pork products (you see on an ingredient label):

- Bacon
- Ham
- Pork Sausage
- Lard
- Pork Fat
- Gelatin
- Animal Shortening
- Mono and Diglycerides (can be made of pork depending on the supplier)
- Lecithin (can be made from pork depending on the supplier)

Increases chances of diseases such as:

- Cardiovascular Disease (Heart Disease and Stroke)
- High Cholesterol
- Obesity
- Cancer
- Diabetes
- Arthritis
- Accelerated Aging

Freedom Factor!

If you are not ready to kick meat out of the window completely, there are still a few things you can do. For starters, begin shopping around for unprocessed meat that comes from organic, grass-fed and farm-raised cattle. Make sure that they are listed as being free of antibiotics and growth hormones. If you eat pork, start by cutting pork products out of your diet. When ready, graduate from red meat to white meat. In place of a slab of steak, have a grilled chicken breast. Instead of eating bacon, try turkey bacon. This is a step forward in the right direction.

White Meat

Including Chicken and Turkey

Today, meat is full of antibiotics and growth hormones. They also contain trace amounts of ammonia. These chemicals build up in the body over a lifetime and affect our growth. Aside from this, foods such as fried chicken have their own list of health problems (this is covered in the "Fried Foods" section of this chapter). We can simply avoid worrying about the risk of food poisoning and foodborne illnesses (such as salmonella and intestinal worms) by leaving meat alone.

Unless we are on a small family farm in a foreign country, there is a good chance we will be eating all sorts of chemicals in our meat. All living things are products of their environment and most of the animals that are used in the meat industry are raised in horrible conditions. Even the soil, air, water and food that an animal eats makes a difference.

Though fruits and vegetables in most places in the US are not as nutrient-rich as they were 50 or 100 years ago, supplementing these nutrients by eating meat is actually more harmful than helpful due to what comes along with it (harmful proteins in the body and unhealthy fats that contribute to kidney and heart problems, obesity, etc.)

White meat consumption increases chances of diseases such as:
Cardiovascular Disease (Heart Disease and Stroke)
High Cholesterol
Cancer

When buying meat, we always want to be aware of where it comes from. Unprocessed, organic, free-range, hormone and antibiotic-free chicken and turkey is a good start. When ready, we can phase into only eating fish, which is much lighter on the system. It can very helpful in this transition to do our research on where our fish comes from and what conditions they are raised in. This is important since fish are highly susceptible to toxins in the water.

Halal & Kosher

Meat in other countries is often healthier due to the way it is handled. Today, we can find some of these cultural standards in our own country. You may have seen the symbols below but did not know what they meant. We will review two of them here.

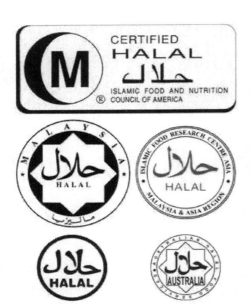

Halal: Meaning *"permissible"* in Arabic. This denotes what is allowed according to Islamic law. In this case, how meat is handled.

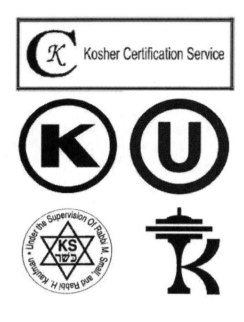

Kosher: Meaning "*fit*" (for consumption) in Hebrew. These are Jewish dietary laws.

Unless you are Muslim or Jewish, as consumers just be aware that both have similar practices when it comes to handling meat.

All Kosher and Halal products are generally healthier due to the following standards:
- They are pork-free (including Kosher gelatin which is often made from fish).
- Animals are not stunned with electrocution before they are killed (lowering the release of toxins into the body).
- The animal is killed immediately, applying a sharp blade to the throat to minimize pain and suffering.
- The animal is inspected to make sure it is free from disease.
- Blood may not be consumed and is therefore completely drained from the meat.

Pareve (or Parve) is under the Kosher umbrella. It means that the foods that they are under do not have meat or dairy products in them (with eggs and fish being the exception). Foods with this label are less likely to be prone to cross-contamination (such as salmonella). Those with dairy allergies can also use this label as a reference.

For healthier options in regard to meat and dairy products, look for these symbols on products you are buying. Also, seek out Kosher, Jewish and Halal markets and restaurants in your area.

Fish

Many people eat fish to get their omega-3 fatty acids. But, we can get that from other grains and supplements such as flaxseed oil without eating fish. The reality is that fish is not the way it used to be. Water pollution, radiation, mercury contamination, fish farming with antibiotics and artificial coloring are just a few factors that play a role into why eating fish is often hurting us more than it is helping us.

What about other kinds of Seafood (crab, shrimp, etc.)?
Most shellfish are bottom feeders. This means that they are the garbage disposals of the ocean. For this reason, I like to call them the "swine of the sea" because, just like pigs, they will eat just about anything they can. For this reason, when we eat shellfish, for example, a whole shrimp, we are eating what is left over in their intestinal tract before they died. Think about that.

Increases chances of diseases such as:
- Cardiovascular Disease (Heart Attack and Stroke)
- Nerve Damage in Brain
- Cancer
- Mental Disorders in children
- Diabetes

Freedom Factor!
When eating fish for nutritional purposes, we can get our protein sources from a plant based diet while getting a good balance of Omega 3 and Omega 6 fatty acids from Flaxseed Oil.

If you are not ready to let go of fish, there are a few important things to consider. Large fish such as tuna, cod, halibut, shark and king mackerel are high in mercury, which is poisonous to the human body. Basically, any fish that eats other fish has higher levels of mercury in them, which is why we should avoid the larger ones. Eat sushi in moderation, since most sushi is made with larger fish such as these. Try eating more catfish and salmon and less shellfish. Tilapia in the United States is what is referred to as "frankenfish." Actually, tilapia in other countries looks nothing like the tilapia here. This is because they are farm-raised and genetically modified to grow faster. Change your diet from farm-raised fish to wild-caught fish. This is a good way to avoid fish that are fed antibiotics, growth hormones and food coloring. Also, be aware of what part of the world it comes from. Many bodies of water are now experiencing high levels of nuclear radiation and mercury poisoning due to pollution. It is important to do our research on where these fish come from and how it is handled before buying it.

Smoked Food

Inhaling smoke from a fire is not the only way that it can harm us. Eating smoked meats and vegetables on a regular basis can actually lead to negative health effects. Smoked foods are considered carcinogenic (cancer-causing). This is because the actual smoke itself has toxic chemicals that are absorbed by the food. Barbecue is a staple in our country and is practiced around the world. For many of us, it is a way of life. However, grilled meat can also be carcinogenic when the outside of the meat is charred. This is because charring food creates certain compounds that are linked to cancer. However, when choosing between smoked or grilled food, grilling is a healthier option.

Rice

Other than wheat, rice is a staple food in most cultures around the world. It is an affordable way to feel full while eating something with it. However, white rice is stripped of most of its nutrients before it gets to you and is a big culprit in digestive issues. Rice basically turns into glue in your intestines and makes it more difficult for our bodies to take in nutrients.

Freedom Factor!
There are a variety of healthier grains (which will be discussed shortly) that can replace rice. Avoid plain white rice. Basmati rice is the next best step. Brown rice is metabolized much better in the body because of its fiber content. Try organic black rice as well. Remember, these grains are best when soaked for 12-25 hours.

Wild rice is not actually a grain (like other rice) but a type of tall grass that is best when soaked or sprouted and then steamed for 5-10 minutes. It is also very filling! Once we start eating other grains, we will find that we will not need rice as a staple in our diet.

Eating excess amounts of rice increases chances of diseases such as:
- Diabetes
- Decrease in Mental Activity
- Constipation

118

Sugar

Sugar, or as many of us would like to call it "Sugar Crack," is one of the most addictive additives we consume today. We think everything tastes better when there is sugar in it. When we start eating something with sugar in it, we crave more. Try not touching sugar or anything with sugar in it for a week. Our bodies will most likely go through the same withdrawal symptoms that someone would go through if they were in rehab. Sweats, irritability, insomnia, headaches, the works. It is an addicting additive.

Sugar, as a sweetener comes from the sugarcane. These sugarcane stalks are chopped down and the juice is extracted mechanically. The product of this is what we call cane juice (which is actually very healthy and even safe for diabetics). It is then boiled off until it turns into a thick, sticky syrup. At this point, it can be filtered and ground into what is known as sucanat, panela, jaggery, or rapadura (each name is simply from a different language and means the same thing). This is the least processed form of sugar on the market and contains all kinds of nutrients, vitamins and minerals. It also processes slower in the body, meaning that it will not spike your blood sugar in the same way that other sugars do.

If it is not turned into sucanat, this sticky mass of evaporated sugar cane juice is spun so that the solid sugar crystals are separated from the sticky substance, which we know as molasses. Molasses is packed with minerals including iron (which is great for those who have anemia). However, you do not get these minerals when you eat white sugar. At this point, it is known as raw cane sugar or turbinado sugar, which is still brown because it contains hints of molasses. Common white sugar is processed, and bleached using charcoal made from cow bones. Common "brown" sugar is simply white sugar with molasses added to it and is no healthier than white sugar. Unless it is organic, the majority of sugar can contains pesticides and has been genetically modified as well.

Many other foods have sugar in them, including fruit. Fruit has natural sugar in it (called fructose), but it comes in a complete package of fiber, enzymes and antioxidants that balance it out. If you buy fructose as a sweetener, it no longer has those things to balance it. On another note, we all know how important Vitamin C is for our immune system. Well, sugar lowers the amount of Vitamin C in your body by replacing it. When sugar goes into the body, Vitamin C is pushed out. This is also how eating too much sugar can make us sick. The bottom line is that a little sugar is okay. However, the more cane sugar we add to our food and drinks, the worse off we are, no matter what form it comes in.

Increases chances of diseases such as:
- Diabetes
- Obesity
- Weakened immune system
- Liver Disease
- Heart Disease
- Insomnia
- Decrease in Mental Activity
- Anxiety
- Depression
- Dementia
- Reproductive Issues in Women

The problem with agave, artificial sweeteners and other sugar substitutes is that they are highly processed and take a toll on our bodies. Some of these are created in a laboratory from chemicals that we would never eat. Simply because they are low in sugar and do not spike your insulin levels does not mean that they are better for us. This includes aspartame, sucralose (Splenda), aspartame (Equal/NutraSweet), saccharin (Sweet'N Low), xylitol, agave and stevia. All of the ingredients named are either artificial sweeteners or sugar substitutes. None of them are better options in place of sugar. Many of them have been known to cause digestive issues and increase the chances of diseases such as cancer, liver and kidney failure. For this reason, it is important to avoid "Diet" drinks and "Sugar-Free" foods and drinks completely. Coconut sugar is a great option. However, it should be used in moderation due to the unethical practice of cutting down whole coconut trees for mass production.

A few natural sweeteners that can be used in moderation include:
- Organic Dates
- Raw and locally farmed Honey
- Raw sugar cane juice
- Maple sugar/organic Grade B Maple syrup
- Panela, Jaggery, Rapadura, Sucanat (least processed form of sugar, full of nutrients, better for blood sugar levels than other cane sugars)
- Organic Turbinado Sugar (second least processed form of sugar)

Honey

Our common store bought honey is mass produced, overly processed and heated at high temperatures doing away with all of the health benefits that honey is touted to have. This honey is just as harsh on the body as sugar.

Freedom Factor!
Raw local honey is your best bet. 100% raw and unfiltered honey is solid at room temperature and has medicinal properties. Not only this, but it tastes amazing!

Eggs

Imagine living on a farm and owning chickens. 5 of them are hens (females who can lay eggs). All 5 of them lay eggs, leaving them with 5 eggs. They eat two and hope the other 3 hatch so that there can be more chickens on the farm. This means they will not have any eggs to eat for days if not weeks. That is the way it goes! Today, we eat way more eggs than normal. Not to mention the growth hormones and antibiotics that are now end up in most of our eggs accumulate in our bodies as well. Things simply are not the same anymore. Even "cage-free" eggs are not what you think they are. Those chickens are not running around happily in a field somewhere. They are all stuffed into the same building, nearly stacked on top of one another. An omelet might be a great way to start the day, but not if it leads to feeling worse later.

Eggs increase the chance of diseases such as:
- Heart Disease (from high blood pressure and cholesterol)
- Obesity
- Eczema
- Asthma
- Faster Aging
- Diabetes
- Sinus Congestion

126

Fried Foods

Just about every culture in every part of the world fries something in oil, grease or lard to make it taste better. The reality of it is that it *does* make it taste better. However, the real question you might want to ask yourself is, "Would I like it if it was not fried and well-seasoned?" If not, maybe you should ask yourself why you are eating it and not something else. Frying anything changes it into something that the body does not recognize as food. Most fried foods that we eat are carcinogenic, which means they are proven to cause cancer. Yet, fried foods are still eaten regardless, because it's all about the taste, right? Wrong. It is tough to enjoy anything when you feel bad.

Eating fried foods increases chances of diseases such as:
- Diabetes
- Heart Disease
- High Blood Pressure
- High Cholesterol
- Obesity
- Cancer (Prostate)
- Acne
- Depression
- Gastrointestinal Issues (IBS, Acid Reflux)

Freedom Factor!

This is a process. We can start cleaning up our diets by modifying *how* we prepare our food and eventually eliminating the food from our diet completely. For example, if we eat fried chicken, then ditch the deep fryer, and go to grilling, then to baking, then eliminating the meat overall. We will find that the less we do to modify the flavor of these things, the less we will feel addicted to them and the easier it will be to eliminate it from our diet completely.

These are examples of how you can take steps in the right direction:

1. Change the oil used to prepare fried food to a healthier alternative (e.g. change bacon fat to coconut oil)
2. Try pan frying instead of deep frying
3. Oven fry food by coating it in a batter and oil and baking it on high temperature
4. Eating roasted or grilled meat and vegetables
5. Baking or boiling meat in a broth instead of cooking it in grease

Salty Snacks

Have you ever gone through a big bag of potato chips in one sitting? Well we are all guilty at one time or another falling prey to the "snack attack". We eat way too much salt and usually crave crunchy, salty snacks like chips and popcorn when we are feeling nervous and anxious. Not to mention, we eat these things unconsciously, usually late at night, while watching TV, as if we are eating a bag of air. It's comforting, but it will not take away your anxiety. Commercial iodized salt or "table salt" or "iodized salt" is bleached with cyanide, aluminum and bleach. I doubt you have ever considered eating any of those things. These small quantities add up over a lifetime and can have a serious affect our internal organs.

This is why sea salt is considered healthier. It has not been tampered with as much. Many foods naturally taste salty or spicy, but our taste buds are overloaded with so much salt, we can barely appreciate the natural flavors of the vegetables that grow on our land. All in all, too much salt is never a good thing, especially white salt.

MSG (or Monosodium Glutamate), used in a lot of Asian cuisine, is popular for its savory and salty flavor. However, it causes severe allergies, migraines, brain damage and disorders of the nervous system. Make sure to look out for this ingredient on food labels and always ask for no MSG when dining out at Asian restaurants.

Increases chances of diseases such as:
- High Blood Pressure (hypertension)
- Osteoporosis (weakened bones)
- Cancer (Stomach)
- Obesity
- Heart Disease

Ingredients that will bring out the saltiness out of your food:
- Lemon/lime
- Onion powder
- Kelp flakes
- Sundried tomatoes (soak them and use the juice or the tomatoes interchangeably)

Himalayan sea salt is one of the healthiest forms of salt because of its mineral content. We end up using less of this salt than others to get the flavor we want out of our food because it packs more of a punch. Combine it with one of the ingredients listed above and we have a recipe for success!

Dairy

We are the only species that drinks the milk from another animal. But, cow's milk is meant for calves. Our bodies are not meant to digest cow's milk and this explains dairy allergies and lactose intolerance. Now, cows are pumped with growth hormones so that they will produce more milk and injected with antibiotics so that they will not get sick and infect the milk. They are also fed with foods full of pesticides. This means that growth hormones, pesticides and antibiotics have gotten into our milk and our bodies. I have always wondered why each generation is so much taller than the other and I would say this is a contributing factor. Not to mention that pus from these cows leeches into the milk as well.

Then, the milk is pasteurized so that it kills all the harmful bacteria, which makes it lasts longer on the shelves. This also kills all the helpful enzymes that supposedly make milk good for the body. What about Calcium? Where would I get it if I do not drink milk? Dark leafy green vegetables (such as kale and spinach) contain high amounts of calcium as well as many fruits, nuts and grains. And we do not have to eat a boatload of it to get the necessary amount of calcium in your diet.

Do not get me wrong, this does not mean that I condone using goat's milk or eating goat cheese. But, it has not been tampered with nearly as much as cow's milk and this would be a step forward if you are making the switch. Furthermore, various goat cheese manufactures even add a hint of cow's milk in their cheese, so you have to really read the labels.

List common dairy products:

- Milk
- Anything with the word "Casein" (Rennet Casein, Potassium Caseinate, etc.)
- Anything with the word "Whey" (Whey Protein, etc.)
- Anything with the word "Butter" (Butter Fat, Butter Solids, Buttermilk, etc.)
- Dry Milk Powder
- Condensed Milk / Evaporated Milk
- Ghee or Paneer (often used in Indian cuisine)
- Cheese (unless it is specified as Dairy Free)
- Custard
- Coffee Creamers
- Yogurt
- Nougat
- Whipped Cream

Watch out for carrageenan gum in milk substitutes. Carrageenan gum on its own is simply Irish moss, a kind of sea algae, used to thicken sauces and more. However, carrageenan gum used in commercial products is processed to the point where it is harmful to the body. The biggest side effect is that it produces inflammation in the intestines. This is why it is important to find dairy-free products without carrageenan gum in them.

Increases chances of diseases such as:

- Obesity
- Cardiovascular Disease
- Cancer (Breast, Prostate)
- Diabetes
- Weakened immune system
- Reproductive Problems
- Kidney Disease
- Asthma
- Eczema

Freedom Factor!

There are dozens of milk substitutes on the market today. Examples of these are almond milk, rice milk, flax milk, hazelnut milk, macadamia nut milk and coconut milk. We can find these at our local grocery store or we can easily make them at home using a high-powered blender. Coconut oil is a great substitute for butter. Dairy free and soy free butter, whipped cream, and cream cheese can also be found in many stores.

Caffeine

I will admit, I am a sucker when it comes to a cup of Persian tea, hot cocoa or coffee. But, it is addictive and I usually have some side effect after drinking it. Whether it is the jitters, trouble focusing, insomnia or frequent trips to the bathroom, the end result is rarely what I wish it would be. Caffeine naturally exists in many things and it is all over the world. Generally, it is either coffee or tea and both of them have their positive and negative effects on the body. Yes, coffee is a great antioxidant, which would help fight aging and cancer. However, most of these antioxidants are destroyed after they are roasted and sit around for a while. Energy drinks have ridiculous amounts of caffeine in them and cause damage to the body over time. Another issue is that most of us drink our caffeinated beverages with a lot of sugar, which makes things worse. Either way, if we already have health concerns, it may be better to consider taking caffeine out of our diets to see how we feel.

Though energy drinks may give us a quick boost of energy, they are more harmful than drinking excess amounts of caffeine. They are high in artificial sweeteners, food colors and preservatives. Also, coffee that contains excess amounts of added ingredients such as taurine can cause strokes, seizures, high blood pressure and heart disease.

Just like any drug, consuming unnatural energy drinks and excess amounts of caffeine wears off over a period of time. Our tolerance will go up and we will need more to get the boost that we are used to. However, the effects of natural ingredients that boost our energy will never wear off. Examples of these are wheatgrass, ginger juice and spirulina. Ingredients such as these boost our energy because of the natural minerals, vitamins, enzymes and antioxidants they contain.

Excess caffeine increases chances of diseases such as:
- Hypertension (high-blood pressure)
- Heart Attack
- Arthritis
- Incontinence (in women)
- Infertility (in women)
- Insomnia
- Indigestion
- Headache/Migraine
- Anxiety
- Depression
- Osteoporosis

Coffee

Although coffee has antioxidants, they are usually roasted and washed out. By the time the coffee gets to our cups and we add a bunch of milk or creamer and sugar to it, we end up drinking a cup of caffeinated sugar instead of a healthy drink full of energy-boosting antioxidants. The only people I know who are old and look young but still drink coffee are the ones who take a small cup of it, freshly ground and black (strong with no sugar or cream). Most of these people are from cultures where their coffee is freshly roasted (something that is a rarity here). Regardless, coffee is a big thing here. However, there are healthy substitutes out there that give us the energy and flavor we need without sacrificing our morning ritual. There are many companies out there that even make coffee substitutes with healthier ingredients (the kind of ingredients that prolong our lives).

Invest in a juicer and watch your coffee maker become obsolete.
- Juice a thumbs length of ginger, one lemon and mix with a hint of cayenne pepper (if you are feeling adventurous) to get a lasting pick-me-up. Not only will it wake up the body, it will clear the sinuses and reduce inflammation. (Those of us who suffer from low blood pressure should not drink ginger juice as it naturally lowers blood pressure)
- To oxygenate the blood, juice any dark leafy green vegetables (chard, spinach, kale, broccoli, etc.) along with a cucumber and a hint of ginger. Have as is or stir in a teaspoon of wheatgrass powder for an energy boost.

138

Carbonated Beverages

"Pop", "Soda", "Soda Pop", whatever we want to call it, carbonated beverages have been a staple in our modern diet. Many of us drink more carbonated beverages than we drink water. We drink it when we are thirsty, after we exercise, while watching TV and during any other daily activity. For starters, carbonated drinks do not rehydrate the body like water does. When we drink something like this when we are thirsty, we are putting our bodies under stress due to dehydration. Also, unless we are drinking plain tonic water (which most of us do not), we are drinking a bunch of sugar, artificial food coloring, and caffeine. One of the common preservatives in carbonated drinks is high fructose corn syrup, a sweetener that has all the negative effects of corn and sugar combined. Certain dark sodas leech the calcium out of your bones, which, in turn, weakens them.

Freedom Factor!
Try kombucha tea or other fizzy drinks that are made with probiotic cultures. Drinks in this category will boost our energy, improve digestion and boost our immune system.

White Potatoes

All potatoes are 100% carbs and starch. They truly have barely any nutritional value whatsoever. Whatever amount of nutrition potatoes have is usually cooked to death in a deep fryer or microwave. I call potatoes "the filler food." It is great for when we want to get full faster, especially when we are on a budget. Not to mention, they are a quick fix. Just pop a potato in the microwave or run to our nearest fast food joint, get an order of French fries and "*Presto!*" we have something to hold us over until we can get our hands on some "real food."

There are two big problems with eating potatoes. The first is that they inevitably lead to constipation and a diminished elimination of waste. This equals a backup of toxins in the body. Secondly, if we are trying to do anything productive throughout our day, forget it, potatoes are extremely high on the glycemic index. In other words, our blood sugar levels will go up, and then crash.

Ever wondered why we feel sleepy after eating a baked potato or a plate of fries? This is due to the fact that potatoes turn into sugar almost as soon as they enter our bodies. As we know, sugar gives us energy and eventually makes us tired. These sugars are then stored in the body as fat. Also, potatoes are like pesticide sponges. So, unless our potatoes are 100% organic, those harmful chemicals are basically impossible to wash off. These are important factors to consider when buying potatoes.

Increases chances of diseases such as:
- Diabetes
- Obesity
- Constipation
- Irritable Bowel Syndrome
- Joint Pain
- Kidney Disease

Freedom Factor!
Sweet potatoes are full of cancer-fighting and anti-aging phytochemicals. They also help reduce inflammation. They can be baked and eaten alone or used in recipes just like other potatoes. Be conscious though, sweet potatoes are starchy root vegetables and too much of these can still weaken our digestive system.

Bananas

If we want to lose weight, have asthma, eczema, or hay fever symptoms, we want to avoid bananas. They cause inflammation and mucus in the body. Especially since most of them are genetically modified and mass-produced. Not to mention, unless they are native to our soil, they are not as nutrient dense or flavorful as they could be.

Bananas increase the chance of diseases such as:
- Obesity
- Asthma
- Eczema
- Diabetes
- Tooth Decay
- Hay fever
- Constipation
- Gastrointestinal Issues (gas)
- Migraines
- Depression

Freedom Food!
Avocados contain more potassium than bananas and can easily be added to smoothies or salads. Not to mention, they are full of heart-healthy fats and keep us full for a long time. Try using a ripe avocado in place of salad dressing. Mashing it up into a guacamole-like sauce with a squeeze of lemon or balsamic vinegar can add a creamy texture to salads and pastas. Avocados are a great addition to any meal.

144

Pasteurized Juice

Store bought juice is pasteurized and stored over extended periods of time where it loses its cancer prevention and anti-aging chemicals. Most juice we buy is often more water and sugar than it is fruit juice. It usually has added sugar, high fructose corn syrup or another artificial sweetener. Most juice contains pesticides (unless it is organic) and comes from genetically modified fruits and vegetables as well. Not only this, but most companies also add artificial flavors, food coloring and artificial preservatives to their beverages while touting the words "made from real fruit juice" on the front of their containers.

The amazing thing is that fruit juice registers in the body as sugar and spikes our insulin levels. Many of us drink juice when we are thirsty, tired or getting sick, but what we do not know is that we are often compromising our health by barraging our bodies with excess amounts sugar. Generally, what the body is really craving is water, not juice.

Store-bought Juice Increases chances of diseases such as:
- Diabetes
- Obesity
- Depression
- Dehydration
- Acid Reflux

Freedom Factor!
Invest in a juicer and drink fresh juice. This way, we get all of the nutrients out of it. Some stores also sell fresh squeezed juice. Just be careful to check the label of when it was made.

For a refreshing alternative, try these options:

- **Coconut water** (without sodium metabisulfite) - full of electrolytes and minerals such as magnesium and potassium to reverse dehydration
- **Fresh pressed sugar cane juice** – alkalizes the body, cleanses the urinary tracts and balances insulin levels (which means it is even safe for people with type 2 diabetes)
- **Fruit-infused spring water** – chop up a citrus fruit and let it set in a container of spring water overnight to add a hint of flavor to your drinking water

Tap Water

Throughout the United States, tap water is contaminated with hormones and pharmaceuticals, which alter our mental state.

Some examples are:
- Chlorine
- Chloride
- Fluoride
- Lead
- Arsenic
- Harmful bacteria (including traces of fecal matter)
- Cyanide

Our bodies are resilient machines so most of us are not going to fall over and die after drinking a glass of tap water. However, the long-term effects mentioned above are not to be taken lightly. Consequently, fluoride dumbs down our intuitive abilities by calcifying (creating a hard shell over) the pineal gland, which is located in the brain and also known as our "third eye." This also disrupts the biological rhythm of the body and can lead to many issues including insomnia and depression.

If we are going to drink tap water and cannot afford a tabletop water distiller, then boiling it, letting it cool and running it through a household water filter afterwards will help get rid of some of the bacteria and heavy minerals. However, our best bet is to purchase distilled or spring water.

Drinking Fluoridated Water Increases chances of diseases such as:
- Cancer (colon, bladder)
- Diabetes
- Kidney Stones
- Heart Disease (Heart Attack)
- Insomnia
- Depression
- Asthma
- Pneumonia
- Reduced Mental Capacity (Senility)
- Premature Aging
- Kidney Disease
- Osteoporosis
- Arthritis
- Dental Decay
- Infertility

Freedom Factor!
Try to minimize the use of bottled water. Unless it is glass, chemicals from the plastic bottle will leech into your water. This can cause issues in the long run including effects on mental health and our reproductive organs. Instead, look up a place that sells distilled or alkaline water by the jug and take our own glass jugs with us.

Almost all ice comes from fluoridated tap water. Make your own ice by pouring purified/spring water into an ice tray and letting it freeze.

Two Machines You Can Buy For Long-Term Use:
- Tabletop Water Distiller
- Fluoride Water Filter

Canned Foods

BPA (or Bisphenol A) is a harmful chemical often found in the lining of aluminum cans, tin cans and plastics. This chemical leeches into our food and builds up in our system over years of eating canned foods. Also, drinks (especially bottled water) sold in thin plastic bottles leech out plastic chemicals (including BPA) into our beverages. This is why it is important to avoid drinking store-bought water out of thin plastic bottles.

To remedy this issue, purchase BPA Free containers or glass bottles. You may also look for food and liquids in cartons since they are not commonly lined with BPA. Consuming any canned or plastic-bottled products on a long-term basis can lead to life-threatening diseases.

BPA increases chances of diseases such as:
- Cardiovascular Disease
- Diabetes
- Cancer (breast, prostate)
- Neurological Disorders
- Obesity
- Infertility
- Weakened Immune System

150

Artificial Ingredients

We are eating and drinking more artificial food dyes than we ever did in the late 1900's. Artificial food coloring is in everything these days. Examples are vitamins, medicines, bread, pickles, and even on the outside of oranges to make them look riper. Most of the major companies that make the processed food that we consume have taken artificial food coloring, flavors and preservatives out of many of their products in the UK, due to studies that have shown that artificial food coloring is linked to a variety of disorders including ADHD. When reading a label, keep in mind that any color on the ingredient list with a number next to it is most likely artificial and therefore harmful to our health (e.g. something labeled with FD&C Yellow no. 5 or Red no. 40).

Here are some examples of safe food coloring that may be found on an ingredient label:
- Carotenes (such as beta carotene, which makes carrots orange)
- Annatto (a seed from South and Central America)
- Beet
- Capsanthin (an extract of paprika)
- Black Currant Extract

Below is a list of Artificial Preservatives you want to avoid:

- TBHQ - can cause nausea and vomiting
- Polysorbate (60, 65 or 80) - can cause infertility
- BHT - can lead to liver and kidney failure
- BHA - Carcinogenic (cancer-causing)
- Nitrate or Nitrite (e.g. Sodium Nitrate) - carcinogenic
- Sodium Benzoate - Carcinogenic
- Sulfites - can cause allergic reactions and asthma

A few healthy, natural preservatives include:

- Ascorbic Acid (Vitamin C)
- Grapeseed Extract
- Rosemary Extract

Artificial Flavors

Chemically made artificial flavors are known to cause problems in the human body such as brain tumors, cancer, nausea, seizures, depression, severe allergies, kidney problems and high blood pressure. Unless the word "natural" is before a flavor listed on an ingredient list, it is most likely artificial.

Artificial Food Additives Increases chances of diseases such as:

- Cancer
- Infertility
- Depression
- ADHD
- Tumors
- Kidney Failure
- Liver Disease
- High Blood Pressure
- Hay fever
- Asthma
- Diabetes

"But, It's Natural!"

Just because the label says that it is "natural" does not mean it is healthy. Companies throw this word around because it sells. Think about this. Would we eat our table? This sounds like an absurd question, right? However, our table is made of natural wood. So, why not? Some companies put wood pulp in our food and call it "cellulose" while touting that it is a "natural" ingredient. Would we eat wood just because it is "natural"? Of course not! So, we should not trust everything we see. We must do our research first. If the ingredient label only says "natural flavors," it may be because those ingredients are not things we would like to eat.

Below are a few unhealthy "natural" ingredients we might read on a label:

- **Confectioner's Glaze (aka Shellac or Lac Resin)** – The coating on chewing gum and hard candies that makes them shiny. This comes from the secretion of beetles in East Asia.

- **Natural Raspberry Flavor (aka Castoreum)** – Comes from the anal secretions of beavers.

- **L-Cysteine (aka L-Cys or L-Cysteine Hydrochloride)** – Used to enhance the flavor in pizza, crackers, meat and vegetarian meat flavored products. Also used to give a "fresh-baked" texture to processed breads, bagels, cupcakes and other baked goods. This product is made from hog hair, human hair or duck feathers. (Look for the vegan option, as this is a natural amino acid)

- **Cellulose** – This is used as a filler in processed meat products, muffins, waffles, pancakes, ice cream and much more. Cellulose is made from wood pulp and is indigestible by the human body.

- **Caramel Color** – Often used in baked goods, soft drinks, sauces, seasonings, candies, medicines and alcoholic beverages. This is created in a laboratory and can be carcinogenic (cancer causing) with long-term use.

Cooking Oils

Not all oils are created equal. It is important to know that many oils improve our health while others can be of a detriment to it. Some contain healthy fats while others contain the fats that will clog our arteries. When shopping for oils, always look for ones labeled "organic," "cold-pressed" and "expeller-pressed." This means that harmful chemicals were not used to extract the oil from the seeds and that they have not been exposed to high heat so they still contain most of their nutrients. Here is a list of oils to use and ones to avoid.

COOK WITH THESE:
- **Coconut Oil** - Great for desserts and has a high smoke point (see explanation of "smoke point" below).
- **Avocado Oil** - Has a rich flavor and high smoke point.
- **Macadamia Nut Oil** - Has a nutty flavor and high smoke point. High in healthy fats which help cardiovascular health.
- **Palm Fruit Oil** – Can be used in cooking (high smoke point). Balanced in saturated and unsaturated fats (50/50) and regulates cholesterol. Use sparingly as it can become acid-forming in excess.

Smoke Point:
When an oil has a high "smoke point" it means that we can cook it at a higher heat without it burning and becoming acidic. Olive oil has a low smoke point and should only be used as is (as opposed to being used to fry food). Coconut oil has a higher smoke point and is great for sautéing and pan-frying.

LOW OR NO HEAT:

- **Olive Oil** - To get the most nutrients and flavor out of this one, using extra virgin (unrefined) olive oil in our salads, soups and more is a great option. Best when not exposed to high heat due to its low smoke point.
- **Flaxseed Oil** - Best when refrigerated and not exposed to heat. High in healthy fats (omega-3's).
- **Sesame Oil** - Best when not exposed to high heat (avoid in excess because of its unhealthy fat content).
- **Walnut Oil** - Best when not exposed to heat (due to its low smoke point). Great in salads.

AVOID:

- **Palm Kernel Oil** – Not to be confused with "Palm Fruit Oil". High is saturated fat which clogs the arteries.
- **Canola Oil** – Almost all canola oil made in the United States is genetically modified, which is why it is best to avoid this oil.
- **Soybean Oil** – Highly inflammatory and acid-forming. Main ingredient in vegetable oil.
- **Corn Oil** – Weakens the liver and increases allergy symptoms.
- **Vegetable Oil** - Contains a mixture of corn and soybean oil.
- **Peanut Oil** – Extracted from peanuts which are an allergen.
- **Grapeseed Oil** – Usually extracted with harmful chemicals
- **Sunflower Oil** – Best to be consumed raw and unrefined or simply avoided because of its unhealthy fat content.
- **Safflower Oil** – Raises the chance of kidney failure and heart disease.
- **Fish Oil** – Though high in healthy omega-3 fatty acids, the body cannot digest this oil. Try flaxseed oil instead.

It is important to research the oils that we are using to know which one is best for the dish we are making. Look out for these oils when reading ingredient labels on pre-packaged foods. It is also helpful to store our oils in the refrigerator to maintain their health-giving properties and to keep them from going rancid.

Preparing food with the wrong oils increases chances of diseases such as:

- Heart Disease
- Cancer
- Depression
- Arthritis
- Diabetes
- Cardiovascular Disease
- Hay Fever (allergy symptoms)
- Kidney Failure
- Liver Disease
- Kidney and Gallstones

Fast Food

Throw together the downsides of eating meat, fried food, excess sugar, excess salt, artificial flavors, artificial sweeteners, artificial food coloring, preservatives, genetically modified, wheat, white potatoes, corn and pesticide-sprayed food and what we get is fast food. Even if we pick the "healthy" items on the menu, if we are lucky, we only get half of these things. Fast food wrappers do not come with ingredient lists, and even if they did, they are not required to name everything they put in their food. So, we do not know what we are getting. Here are some of the dangers of eating fast food:

Increases chances of diseases such as:
- Obesity
- Diabetes
- High Blood Pressure
- Cardiovascular Disease (heart attack, stroke)
- Gastrointestinal Issues
- Constipation
- Skin Conditions (acne, eczema)
- Depression
- Migraine/Headache
- Kidney Disease
- Asthma
- Sleep Apnea
- Osteoporosis
- Decreased Dental Health (cavities, gingivitis)
- Poor Mental Health

160

Peanuts

Unlike other nuts, which grow on trees, peanuts are actually beans. These beans grow in the ground and are exposed to eight times the amount of toxic fungicides and insecticides than other nuts and beans. This dramatic increase in toxic chemicals is one of the main reasons why so many people have developed peanut allergies over the years. Also, the majority of the mass produced peanuts that we consume have been grown and processed in manufacturing plants. Peanuts naturally contain fungus. Our bodies can tolerate this fungus in small amounts. The problem is that when peanuts are produced in these shaded, moist production plants, this fungus flourishes. The fungi produces a cancer causing chemical called aflatoxin, which over time takes a toll on our internal organs. Those who have peanut allergies are not allergic to the peanuts themselves but the aflatoxins. These toxins spread to anything else that is made in these plants. This causes symptoms such as hay fever and severe allergic reactions in many people. Due to their toxic content and high level of phytic acid, peanuts and peanut butter should be avoided.

Freedom Factor!
To reduce the excess amounts of toxic insecticides and fungicides, buy organic peanut butter and refrigerate it to reduce the production of aflatoxins. Organic almond butters and sunflower butters are even healthier options. These should not be eaten in excess either. This especially applies to cashew butter since cashews are acid-forming. Try eating other raw, sprouted nuts, such as almonds and brazil nuts, which are high in nutrition and easier to digest. We can even soak or sprout raw nuts at home and store them in the fridge for up to five days. Put them in a food dehydrator to give them that crunch we crave. Doing this will also make them last longer.

Breath Fresheners

Most chewing gum, breath mints, breath sprays and other breath fresheners are full of harmful and unnatural food dyes, sweeteners and preservatives.

Freedom Factor!
Nature has provided us with everything we need including ways to freshen our breath. For centuries, people have chewed on herbs and seeds after meals that would not only make their breath smell better, but would assist with digestion, whiten their teeth and ward off any unwanted diseases. A few example of these are listed below:

- Xylitol-based gums
- Fresh basil
- Mint
- Spearmint
- Rosemary
- Parsley
- Fennel
- Anise
- Licorice
- Cloves
- Cinnamon
- Cardamom
- Coriander

164

Alcoholic Beverages

Since most alcoholic beverages are made from fermented hops, they contain wheat. Which, as we know, has numerous negative effects on the body. Not only do they take a toll on our liver but they also register in our bodies as sugar, which in turn causes a buildup of fat in the body. Ever heard of a "beer belly"? This is where it comes from.

What about red wine? Here is the long answer. All of this rave about how a glass of red wine a day fights cancer and can keep us from aging as quickly is a marketing scheme. The antioxidants and enzymes that achieve these positive, anti-aging and immune boosting effects are in the red grapes. In other words, this can just as easily be achieved with a glass of grape juice. The calories in wine can help lead to obesity if not done in moderation.

On an emotional level, many of us are self-medicating. We drink in order to calm our nerves because we have trouble doing it on our own. This only makes us dependent on alcohol. So, here is the opportunity to put the power back in *your* hands. The truth is when we have a balanced eating lifestyle, our minds, bodies and emotions become balanced as well. In other words, by simply feeding our bodies the right things at the right time, we can easily calm our nerves because we will *feel* balanced. Of course, the way we live our lives (including our daily habits) plays an important role. But, that is for another conversation.

Regular consumption of alcohol increases chances of diseases such as:

- Cancer (Mouth, Throat, Liver, Breast)
- Heart Disease
- High Blood Pressure
- Liver Disease
- Diseased Pancreas (Pancreatitis)
- Pneumonia
- Weakened Immune System
- Obesity
- Diabetes
- Depression

Dried Fruit

Most dried fruit contains sulfites (in the form of Potassium Metabisulfite or Sulfur Dioxide), which are artificial preservatives. These sulfites cause allergic reactions in the body, especially in people with asthma. Many of them also contain table sugar, corn syrup or artificial food coloring.

These additives to dried fruit are the real culprits. Be aware though. Even unsulfured dried fruit contains much more sugar (fructose) than regular fruit and, for this reason, it should be eaten in moderation. Otherwise it can lead to obesity, diabetes and other diseases. Unfortunately, sulfites are not bound to dried fruit. They are often added to condiments such as hot sauces and salad dressings as well as packaged seafood such as dried shrimp and anchovies. Be sure to look out for sulfites when reading ingredient labels.

Sulfites increase chances of diseases such as:
- Asthma
- Migraines
- Hay fever

Freedom Factor!
We want to look for dried fruit that is listed as "sulfur-free" or "unsulfured." Also look for dried fruit that it is free of artificial food coloring and has little or no sugar added. Another option is to invest in a food dehydrator and make homemade dried fruit. For those of us who eat a lot of dried fruit, making our own can be very cost-effective in the long run.

Seasonings
&
Spices

Be careful with when consuming various seasonings and spices. Many commercial producers are putting harmful things in them simply to improve their shelf life and save money.

Many spice mixes, such as seasoning salt, add these ingredients to their products:
- Wheat (to stretch out the product)
- Artificial food coloring (to make it more visually appealing)
- Silicon dioxide / Silica (to keep it from clumping)

The negative health effects of wheat and artificial food coloring have already been discussed. Many people have an allergy to silicon dioxide and it is known to irritate the lungs. Make sure you read the ingredient label of your seasonings before you buy them. It is important to know that all herbs and spices are actually medicinal in nature. When used properly, they can be disease-fighting and anti-aging miracles.

Replace black or white pepper with cayenne pepper. Even though black pepper has its health benefits, it becomes an irritant once it is cooked. This means that it can cause inflammation in the body. Cayenne pepper contains capsaicin, which is used as an over-the-counter pain reliever. Basil is known to reduce inflammation and is a natural antibiotic. Ginger is great for digestion and relieves sinus pain. The fresher our herbs and spices can be, the greater they will work for us. Try buying spices whole, investing in an herb grinder, and grinding them right before adding them to any culinary dishes. Along with their healing properties, fresh herbs also have an amazing flavor! Look out for these flavorful, fresh herbs in various local grocery stores.

Reading Labels

What to keep in mind when shopping around

Avoid products that say things like this under the ingredient list:
- "May contain __(insert food item here)__"
  - (e.g. May contain peanuts)
- "Shared on the same equipment that processes ___"
  - (e.g. Shared on the same equipment that processes peanuts)
- "Processed in the same facility that processes ___"
  - (e.g. Processed in the same facility that processes soy)

When we change our eating lifestyle and remove things from our diet, we want to *completely* eliminate an ingredient from our diet. That means no wiggle room. Otherwise, we may not get the outcome we want and need.

When reading an ingredient label, if we cannot pronounce it, then we probably should not eat it. If the ingredient is not familiar in context, look it up! Even though labels are not as truthful or accurate as they used to be (thanks to bills passed by our government), it is still in our best interest to read labels. Be mindful that ingredients change. Always check the label of a product, even if we have bought it many times before. We never know what we may find.

Processed & Overcooked Foods

How to get the most out of your food

Everything in nature has its natural balance, including food that grows from the earth. When we eat an orange, the sugars in the orange are balanced by the fibers of its fleshy pulp, which contain vitamins, minerals, acids, oils and enzymes that balance themselves in the body. This is the case with any whole food. Every time we cook the life out of something, or process (break down) food, it loses most of these vitamins, minerals and enzymes that bring the balance and all that is left is a plate of sugar, fiber and starch. This is why something like an orange is so healthy when we eat it whole, but when we drink orange juice (or any kind of juice at that) it spikes our sugar levels. There is no balance!

Many foods today are processed to the point that the body does not even recognize it as food (e.g.: TVP or Texturized Vegetable Protein). In that case, we may as well be eating plastic. However, if we do not feel like eating a bowl of plastic, keep reading.

Boiled vs. Steamed veggies

In many cultures, we boil our vegetables until they get nice and tender. Collard greens are a great example of this. To make classic, soul food collards, we simmer collard greens in a pot of water for at least two hours. My aunt would cook them for up to half a day. They may taste good afterwards, but all that is left of them is a bunch sugary starch and fibers. So, instead of getting the benefits from the cancer fighting, anti-aging and energy boosting nutrients in collards, all we get is good taste mixed with low energy and possible constipation.

When it comes to cooking, lightly cooking our food (preferably steaming for 5-10 minutes or lightly braising) is fine. However, if our piece of broccoli went from crunchy and bright green to mushy and dark green or brown, we are cooking the life out of our food (literally). This is a rule of thumb for any kind of food. This is also why it's important that at least 50% of the things you eat are raw and fresh fruits and vegetables. If we can get to 80% raw foods and 20% cooked foods, we are on a roll. If we are feeling adventurous, try doing 100% raw (and soaked) foods for some time and see how we feel. We might be surprised.

When you eat cooked or processed foods, it is already lacking certain nutrients that our bodies are craving, so we are going to want to eat more and more to make up for that. Our country thrives off of selling "convenient" and overcooked, over processed foods and it is too easy to pick up a hamburger, snack cake, french fries, bag of chips or a box of cookies on our way to or from work. One of the reasons (aside from all the sugar, fat, etc.) that we have trouble *not* eating more is because we are barely getting anything out it (nutrient-wise) and our bodies are telling us to eat more in order to compensate. This becomes a never ending cycle and kills our wallets and eventually our bodies.

There is a solution though! When we eat, unprocessed, raw, soaked, or lightly cooked foods in their natural form (e.g.: if a green bean still looks like a green bean and not a brown and fried chip), we will get so much more out of our food (nutrient-wise). This will help end cravings, give us more energy and we will actually find out that we are saving time and money because we are eating and cooking less while feeling much more satisfied. When it comes to comfort food, there is nothing like a piece of fried chicken, a plate of french fries or a bag chocolate chip cookies. Most of us are hooked on those things like a drug, and this is because, in a sense, they are drugs.

Food is medicine and the wrong medicine can be poison.

In an effort to take control of our well-being, starting our own rehabilitation program is a good way to get started on a healthier path. Some of us reading this book are probably be somewhere along the journey, which means we want to make the change. So, we must give ourselves a pat on the back because that alone should be honored. Now, it is time to take the next step forward!

Breakfast Foods

The right way to start your day

Breakfast is touted as the most important meal of the day. How we start our day often sets the course of how it will continue. However, what most of us choose to eat for breakfast tastes better than it feels. Most pancakes, waffles, buttery biscuits and rolls all contain dairy, corn, soy, wheat, artificial preservatives, food coloring along with artificial flavors.

Most of our breakfast cereals stocked on the isle of our local grocery store contain a whole bunch of unhealthy additives including wheat, corn, soy, excess sugar, sugar substitutes, artificial food coloring, artificial preservatives and artificial flavors. Even the breakfast foods in the frozen food section or the pre-made pancake and waffle mixes have these things in them.

I am sure we know people who would eat cereal for breakfast, lunch and dinner if they could. This may even be us! Cereal is addictive because of all the sugar and carbohydrates it contains. However, it barely has any nutrients. Why do we think we feel like taking a nap after breakfast? If anything, these foods throw our bodies more off balance than we think.

To top it off, we add a plate of eggs and bacon to the menu and wash it all down with a glass of milk. Only doing this with the notion that it is a "balanced breakfast" and will make us feel full enough to make it through our day. This is further from the truth then you may know. Protein is the hardest thing for our bodies to break down. So, when we overload on proteins (such as bacon and eggs) first thing in the morning, it puts our bodies in shock, actually making it harder for us to focus for the rest of the day.

WORDS OF WISDOM

Gently awaken your body

Take time to let the body gently wake up in the morning. It is important not to shock the body with caffeine and heavy foods when we first get up. We live in a consumerist society where the motto is "time is money." So, we feel the pressure to rush through everything. However, the most important part of the day is when you first get up. It sets the tone for the rest of the day. If you get up a little earlier and take the time to wake our bodies up with warm liquids such as lemon water, tea or fresh fruit juices and basic smoothies, our bodies and our hearts will thank us. This will help us cleanse our system of toxins and train our nerves to be steady throughout the rest of the day. I like to take two hours before I start my day to do this. Look at the countries with the highest life expectancy. They take their time in the mornings to allow their bodies to wake up. So, we have to give ourselves time and if we do not have the time, we have to make the time.

PART III

Action

Putting knowledge into practice

WORDS OF WISDOM

Your first meal should be light.

Our first meal of the day should be light. We should always wake our bodies up gently. Start off with a freshly made juice, herbal tea or glass of warm lemon water. Then have a bowl of fruit or a fruit smoothie. How we start our day off sets the tone for the rest of the day. So, do we want to feel heavy and rushed or light, open and ready to tackle whatever comes across your path? We have to give ourselves time. It is important to eat how we want to feel.

Breakin' It Down

Soaking and Sprouting

If we have ever eaten sunflower seeds or corn on the cob, we may have realized something very different about these foods than others. This would be that they leave our bodies almost the same way they went in. Whole! This is because our bodies are not set up to fully digest nuts, seeds and grains in their natural state. In reality, they are all seeds.

If we think about it, seeds are protected by an outer layer (called enzyme inhibitors) that allow them to be preserved for years, even centuries. This is so that they can sprout and create new plants when placed in the earth. This also means that all of the nutrients in these seeds are locked away until this outer layer is removed. Soaking our grains, nuts and seeds breaks down the enzyme inhibitors, allowing our bodies to digest them properly and take in more of their nutrients.

We could look at soaking seeds as if we were *tricking* them into growing by placing them in water. As a result, they end up removing their protective layer in order to grow, exposing the life-giving nutrients that were once hidden inside. When we learn to soak our grains before cooking them, we will not only feel better but we will eat less since we are getting more nutrients out of our food.

Seeds, nuts, grains and beans also contain phytic acid. This acid actually blocks calcium, magnesium, zinc and copper in the body. This can cause deficiencies in the body in relation to proper absorption of vitamins and minerals. However, when we soak our grains, this reduces the amount of phytic acid.

Instructions on how to soak your food:

1. Pour purified or spring water (at room temperature) into a large bowl.
2. Stir in a teaspoon of baking soda (per 5 cups of water) or Apple Cider Vinegar to help balance the acidity of the water.
3. Pour in your grains and allow them to sit, uncovered for 12 hours.
4. Pour off the liquid, strain, rinse and repeat steps 1-3.
5. After the second 12-hour period, pour off the liquid, strain, rinse in cold water and your grains are ready to be cooked!

If these are nuts, we can simply eat them as is or place them in a food dehydrator to give them a roasted texture. Placing them in an oven on high heat would cook away much of its nutritional value.

This applies to all seeds, nuts and grains such as lentils, rice, millet, almonds, sesame seeds, beans, whole grain wheat, steel cut oats and more. Planning is our friend. We should do our best to soak what we can overnight. It is best to soak our grains for 24 hours; however, even 12 hours can make a difference.

If we continue to soak our grains, they will begin to sprout (as a seed would underground). When a seed begins to sprout, it splits open, removing its protective layer that once locked away all of its life-giving nutrients. Once a grain begins to sprout, it has transitioned from a seed to a plant, meaning that it has completely unlocked all of its nutrients. This is the healthiest way to eat grains, however, the flavor and texture will vary depending on what it is. For example, most sprouted beans taste like raw vegetables, even when cooked. These are great in salads! The key here is to take our time and explore what works for us. We may be surprised at what we can cook up in your own kitchen.

There are companies that make breads and other baked goods with sprouted grains. Look for these online or at our local health food stores.

The
Bean Dilemma

How to cook beans the right way

Beans and other legumes are staples in the United States and abroad. However, beans, just like any seed, are tough to digest. Beans and other seeds contain phytic acid, which reduces the amount of calcium and iron in the body. Legumes also contain proteins that the body cannot digest.

There are many other options of protein-rich grains, which are much easier on the digestive system (such as millet, quinoa and buckwheat), however, if we are going to eat beans every now and then, we must prepare them properly. To do so, here is a recipe for success:

1. Soak them for 24 hours (following the instructions on soaking grains above)
2. Cook them on low heat for a minimum of 6 hours (the longer, the better)
3. Add foods and herbs that assist in digestion such as fresh ginger, garlic, turmeric, cayenne pepper and okra.
4. Do not combine with starches (such as rice) or other proteins (such as meat)
5. Make sure each meal includes at least 50% raw foods (such as a salad of dark green leafy vegetables).

This does not include canned beans, which contain traces of cancer-causing BPA. Canned beans are cooked and canned. The issue here is that soaking after cooking does not remove phytic acid or any of the proteins in the beans that make them indigestible. This only works if you soak them first. Also, a bag of dry beans is much more affordable than pre-cooked canned or boxed beans.

For reference, below is a short list of legumes:
- Black beans
- Black-eyed peas
- Alfalfa
- Chickpeas
- Fava beans
- Lentils
- Peas
- Green Beans
- Peanuts (yes, they are not nuts, but legumes)
- Soybeans

Side Note: Cocoa and Coffee Are The Pits!
Contrary to popular belief, coffee is not actually bean. Coffee "beans" are made from the seed, or pit, of the coffee fruit, which grows on a coffee tree. The fruits look like cherries. In short, coffee is from the seed of a fruit. Cocoa, which chocolate is made from, is the same as coffee. It is also made from the seeds of a fruit (a cacao pod). For this reason, cocoa "beans" are not beans at all. Keep in mind that both of cocoa and coffee still come from seeds, so the same rules apply. Cacao is already fermented in order for it to be edible, yet coffee is not. This could also explain why cocoa and chocolate are so widely known for their health benefits while coffee is still understood to be acid-forming and unhealthy. The truth is that because coffee is not fermented, it still contains its phytic acid, which is why it tends to promote vitamin and mineral deficiencies.

Fermenting Foods

Boosting digestion and immune health

Just because something ferments does not mean it's no longer good. Fermented foods are great for digestion because they are full of healthy bacteria. We call these healthy bacteria "probiotics." This healthy bacterium also boosts the immune system. Yogurt is a form of fermented milk, which is full of beneficial probiotics. Today, we can find yogurt made from almond milk and even coconut milk. kombucha, made from fermented yeast and sugar, is a drink that has been growing in popularity over the years. When it is homemade and unpasteurized (which most store-bought kombucha is not), this tea is full of healthy probiotics. Originally, cheese was created through a fermentation process, which would make it much easier to digest as well.

What about fermenting other things, such as fruits or vegetables? This is a very popular practice worldwide. Kimchi is fermented cabbage native to Korea and is very similar to sauerkraut in the United States. Pickles can just about be made of any kind of fruit or vegetable such as olives, cucumbers, garlic, plums and cabbage to name a few. Homemade pickles are full of life-giving probiotics. The reason I am saying "homemade" here is because, for safety standards, store-bought pickles are pasteurized (heated until the bacteria dies) and no longer contain the healthy probiotics they are known for.

Chocolate is initially made from fermented cacao beans. Before these beans are fermented, they are actually unsafe for human consumption. Cassava is a very common staple food in Africa, South America and Asia. It is also known as manioc, yucca or tapioca. The cassava root contains natural cyanide and is poisonous to eat until it is fermented and strained. Fermentation removes the cyanide and makes it possible to eat.

How do certain groups of people in other parts of the world eat things like bread and still remain so healthy? The trick is fermentation. Beyond soaking our grains, fermentation takes it a step further. When soaked grains sit for long enough in the right environment, the bacteria in the air, known as yeast, begins to eat away at the grains. If this is allowed to happen long enough, the bacteria actually pre-digests the grains for us, breaking them down to the point where they are much more digestible for humans. Fermenting grains also completely removes phytic acid and turns it into a great source of magnesium, calcium and iron. Those suffering from calcium or iron-deficiencies (including anemia) should keep this in mind.

When we watch something ferment, it begins to bubble. This is exactly how bread was made for centuries before yeast was introduced into the baking process. Bakers would leave their bread out for days (in the right temperature), allowing the grains in their bread to ferment before they were baked. The natural yeast from the air around them would create bubbles in the dough and these bubbles would create air pockets in the bread, making it rise. Once baked, this is what originally gave bread its crispy-on-the-outside yet fluffy-on-the-inside texture. This is also what made bread easier to digest.

The practice of adding brewer's yeast to bread, instead of allowing yeast to naturally occur did not happen until the Industrial Revolution in the mid-19th century. People did not have as much time to cook and therefore needed more food, quickly. Adding commercial yeast shortened the baking process from days to hours and companies were able to make much more money. The only problem with this was that the grains were not given the time they needed to ferment, leaving them almost indigestible. Most of the bread we eat is made this way today. Fermentation is what gives breads such as sourdough and Ethiopian injera their sour taste. It is also what makes them easier to digest, allowing us to soak in much more of the nutrients out of the grains. Many people are now using yeast in even these types of breads in order to produce more of them much more quickly.

Wild fermentation is when the natural yeasts that are floating around in the air come into contact with our food, allowing it to ferment. (This is different from when we add commercial yeast to food to make it ferment) This is how we also get naturally leavened bread.
The word "leaven" means to make dough rise through fermentation. This is done with what we call a "leavening agent," which is another way of saying "something that makes dough rise through fermentation." As discussed earlier, this can be done naturally, over the course of time or much more quickly, using commercial baker's yeast. Naturally leavened bread and baked goods are the healthier option, since the grains actually ferment. Do a search online or at any local health food store to find bread that is naturally leavened. After reading this, we may even be inspired to learn how to bake our own bread.

188

Candida Overgrowth

The cause of many diseases

Our intestines naturally have a yeast in them called "candida" which helps break down what we eat and turn it into nutrients. The right amount of this yeast helps the body without hurting it. However, many of our diets make this candida grow too much and this overgrowth of candida in the body causes all kinds of issues. A few examples of diseases caused by candida overgrowth are:

- Skin Conditions (including Eczema, Psoriasis, Hives, Rashes)
- Asthma
- Indigestion (including acid reflux, constipation and diarrhea)
- Fungal Infections (in skin and nails)
- Yeast Infection
- Severe Hay Fever (allergy symptoms)
- Chronic Joint Pain
- Weakened Immune System

Candida overgrowth can get so bad that it can even get into the bloodstream. This becomes a contributing factor to chronic diseases such as Lupus, Fibromyalgia, Chronic Anemia, and all forms of cancer. The real problem with too much candida in the intestines is that it keeps the body from taking in all of the nutrients of what we eat and drink. In turn, we end up with mineral deficiencies, which weaken the body and the mind.

The good news is that we can reverse this by simply cleaning up our diets. By doing this, our bodies will heal themselves. How do we do this? Simply start by using the information in this book!

Nutritional Yeast

Good or bad?

Nutritional Yeast and Brewer's Yeast do not affect candida because they are "dead" yeasts, so they cannot be processed by candida. However, if we have a toxic buildup of candida in our system, then any kind of yeast (nutritional, brewer's yeast or even naturally-occurring yeasts including kombucha) may make us feel bad. There is no connection between MSG and these yeasts. However, torula yeast and hydrolyzed yeast extract are related to MSG and should be avoided.

Any claims that nutritional yeast is high in vitamins and minerals including Vitamin B12 are false. The reason nutritional yeast contains any vitamins or minerals is because it is "fortified" by the manufacturer. This means they add these *artificial* vitamins in after they pasteurize (cook, kill, dry and grind) the yeast. These artificial vitamins and minerals are not recognized by the body as food. Therefore, ingesting them results in gastrointestinal issues.

It is important to note that all nutritional and brewer's yeasts were created from live probiotic cultures and then heated until the yeast is dead and can no longer grow. In turn, they are not going to improve your health the same way that live probiotics do. The point is when we cleansing or detoxing, we want to avoid adding yeasts to our diets because our bodies are trying to balance out the naturally occurring yeasts that it are already has too much of.

When something is naturally in a food, it processes differently in our bodies. However, when we add it in separately, our bodies can often reject it, because it does not come with the natural balance of fibers, vitamins, minerals, enzymes and amino acids that the natural *whole food* would. This is why I recommend that we avoid supplemental yeast. It is different than a powdered superfood.

Take wheatgrass powder, for example. It is simply wheatgrass that is dried, ground and packaged for consumption. This is very different than the nutritional yeast that is grown from sugar and beet molasses, then killed by heating it to high enough temperatures, dried, ground, fortified with artificial nutrients and then packaged. Over-the-counter nutritional or brewer's yeast is a processed extract.

The beets, sugar, molasses or corn syrup used to create nutritional yeast is often full of pesticides, insecticides and is genetically modified. The trick is that as long as the yeast that these beets, sugar, molasses or corn syrup create is not sprayed with pesticides itself, it can be labeled "organic." The same goes for "non-GMO." So, even though nutritional yeast may be labeled as a "health food," the source of the yeast may not be so healthy.

Allergies & Intolerances

Getting to the root of allergic reactions

There are two thing we must understand when it comes to allergies:

1.) Our bodies already have their own natural defenses to allergy symptoms.
2.) What we eat helps to determine how well our bodies react to allergies in our environment (pollen, dust, etc.).

Growing up, I had severe allergies and, come spring, I was always the first one to be coughing, itching, wheezing and sneezing; without fail. While I was in college, I decided to try eating only uncooked fruits and vegetables and lightly cooked grains (other than wheat). After my first three months of going completely raw/vegan, spring came and the streets were covered in pollen. Well, I was just sure that I was going to start sneezing as soon as I stepped outside. But, something amazing happened. My eyes began to water to clean out the pollen, but they did not itch or burn. My nose did not run or get stuffy. And most of all, I was not sneezing or asthmatic. It was amazing!

The lesson of this experience is that when we take care of our bodies, they will take care of us. The few symptoms that I had (watery eyes or the need to blow my nose every now and then) was simply my body taking care of itself. But, it did not interfere with the quality of my life.

Below is a list of the most common foods that people are allergic to:
- Milk
- Eggs
- Fish
- Shellfish (e.g. Shrimp)
- Tree nuts (e.g. Walnuts)
- Peanuts
- Wheat
- Soy

Looking at the list above, we have to ask ourselves, "Why are so many people allergic to these foods in the first place?" There are two answers to this question. The first is that some of these ingredients were never meant for human consumption. Meaning, our bodies are not set up to digest them. The second is that every one of these ingredients has been tampered with and genetically altered so much over the years that our bodies have built up intolerances to them. Either way, these ingredients are not recognized as food and are therefore, rejected by the human body. As a result, we have to look at alternative options to what we can eat.

The Ultimate Four

Key things to remember

So, let us look at the four key things to remember when choosing what to eat:

- Eating in season (pg. 65)
- Proper food combining (pg. 59)
- Removing inflammatory foods from your diet (pg. 41)
- Replacing these with healthy, nutrient-rich, alkaline and anti-inflammatory foods (refer to alkaline food chart on pg. 48)

Remember these four points when creating new recipes or recreating old ones. Applying these to our eating lifestyle will significantly shift the course of our lives and those around us. It is amazing what a little knowledge can do.

WORDS OF WISDOM

Eat what naturally tastes good.

If we have to cover something up with a bunch of salt, sugar, seasonings or oil and we cannot simply enjoy it as is, maybe we should not be eating it in the first place. For example, we do this with coffee, adding so much cream and sugar that it barely tastes like coffee anymore. We often do the same thing with meat. Many of us cannot eat meat unless it is fried in a deep fryer or covered in sauce. Do not get me wrong. I love well-seasoned food. However, there are so many things to eat that are delicious in their natural state. These are the things we want to be eating.

Freedom Foods

Everything you can eat

In order to free ourselves from unhealthy eating patterns, we need to know what our options are. It is important to know that there are healthy alternatives to all of the foods you are eliminating from your diet. As a guide, I have included an abbreviated list with everything that has been discussed in the previous chapters as well as a sample meal plan. In the following pages, you will find descriptions of some of these ingredients along with easy-to-follow recipes. Feel free to jazz them up. Try something new! Pick something from the list that and try something new! Keep in mind that many companies are beginning to use these healthier ingredients in their products. Keep an eye out for these while shopping online or at a local health food store. The following recipes can inspire us on how to make steps forward along our journey. Feel free to mix and match any of the foods on this list. Get creative and have fun!

FREEDOM FOODS

		Buy Organic
Eat in Season		
½ Gallon of alkalized & room-temperature water a day (or more depending on body weight)		
At least 50% fresh fruits/vegetables [or] Raw or lightly steamed vegetables		
Soak, sprout or ferment all nuts, grains and seeds		
Look for glass containers or plastics & cans labeled **"BPA Free"**		
Anti Inflammatory Foods		
Dark leafy green vegetables, garlic, onion, ginger, turmeric, radishes, citrus fruits, pineapple, berries, peppers, beets, chia seeds, coconut oil		
Alkaline Forming Foods		
[Most] fruits, vegetables, herbs, nuts, seeds, herbal teas		
Protein-Rich Foods		
Millet, quinoa, buckwheat, amaranth, teff, sorghum		
Lentils, chickpeas	Veggie burgers (free of wheat & soy)	Rice, quinoa or buckwheat (soba) noodles
Sweet potatoes (vs. white potatoes)	Avocadoes (vs. bananas)	Unsulphured dried fruit
Breads		
Naturally-leavened (home baked) bread, gluten-free & vegan breads, breads with sprouted grains		
Still Eating Meat?		
Halal & Kosher meats, wild-caught & sustainably farm-raised fish (low on the food chain), baked & oven-fried meat		
Milk & Dairy Substitutes		
[Milk made from] almond, rice, flax, hazelnut, macadamia nuts		
[Soy-free & vegan] cream cheese, butter, whipped cream, coffee creamer		
Caffeine Substitutes		
Wheatgrass, ginger juice, spirulina, guarana, açaí, ginseng, brand-name coffee substitutes		

Beverages	Oils	Sugars	Salts	Seasonings
Fresh Juices	Olive oil	Dates	Himalayan sea salt	Organic herbs, spices & roots
Fresh Smoothies	Walnut oil	Raw & local honey	Black salt	(e.g. fresh basil,
Herbal teas	Coconut oil	Sucunat (aka. Panela,	Kelp flakes	cayenne pepper,
Coconut water	Flaxseed oil	Jaggery)	Lemon/lime (juice or	ginger root, turmeric)
Sugar cane juice	Avocado oil	Turbinado sugar	powder)	
Fizzy probiotic drinks	Sesame oil		Sundried tomatoes	
Kombucha tea	Macadamia Nut oil		(soaked)	
Fruit-infused spring water				

Breath Fresheners

Xylitol-based gums, fresh mint, basil, rosemary, fennel

Vitamin & Mineral Supplements

Vitamins D3, B12, B7 (biotin)

Flaxseed oil (Omega 3 & 6), Kelp (Iodine)

Sample Meal Plan

Water Therapy	Breakfast (light meal)	Lunch (complete meal)	Dinner (light meal)	Sundown/3-4hrs before sleep
30min before breakfast	Herbal tea	Protein-rich grains, etc.	Salad	Herbal tea
	Fresh fruit juice	Raw/Steamed veggies	Light grains	Fresh fruit
	Fruit smoothie	Healthy Starches	Steamed veggies	Leafy green salad
		Veggie Burger/Bean	(little to no	(spinach, chard, etc.)
	Soaked oats	Burger	starches/proteins)	

(Snack in between meals. Snacking is good!)

Millet

Freedom From: Rice, Corn, Wheat and Soy.

Health Benefits: Gluten-free, alkaline in nature, high in protein, reduces migraines, reduces chance of heart attack, gives you energy while barely raising your blood sugar, helps with constipation, feeds healthy bacteria in your gut, easy to digest

Flavor: Millet has a very neutral flavor. With just a dash of salt and oil, it can taste like corn grits. Add a bit of sugar and coconut oil and it tastes like cream of rice or rice pudding.

Consistency: When cooked properly, millet has the consistency of corn grits. When used as flour in baking it adds a wholesome and flaky texture to baked goods. Similar to corn meal.

RECIPE

Millet Grits
2 cups Whole Millet
4 cups Water
2 tbsp. Olive Oil or Coconut Oil
1 tbsp. Dried Oregano
½ tbsp. Dill Seed Powder
1 tbsp. Dried Dill Weed
1 tsp. Sea Salt

Directions:
Soak your millet for 12-24 hours for best results. Add your millet, water, salt and oil to a pot and bring to a boil. Lower to medium-low heat while stirring intermittently for the next 20-30 minutes. While stirring, add your oregano, dill seed powder and dill weed. Remove from heat and let sit with the top on for 10-15 minutes.
Servings: 3-5

Quinoa

Freedom From: Rice, Corn, Wheat and Soy.

Health Benefits: Gluten free and high in protein. Contains all the essential amino acids which means that it can help quickly build protein (including muscle) in the body. Improves heart health. Naturally high in iron, so it helps build blood and remedy iron deficiencies (e.g. anemia). Helps regulate blood sugar.

Flavor: Has a light, nutty flavor but picks up the flavor of anything you combine it with
.

Consistency: Light, fluffy and grainy.

RECIPE

Sweet and Spicy Quinoa
2 cups White Quinoa
4 cups Water
½ cup Dried Cherries (diced)
1 tbsp. Sliced/Slivered Almonds
2 tbsp. Coconut Oil
Cilantro
4 Garlic cloves (chopped)
1 tsp. Curry Powder
1 tbsp. Ground Coriander
½ tsp. Sea Salt
1/8 tsp. Cayenne Pepper
2 Dried Red Chili Peppers (cut in half)
1 tsp. Lime Juice
1 tsp. Cane Sugar
1 Red Onion (diced)

DIRECTIONS:

Before cooking, soak quinoa for 12-24 hours for best results.

Pour you water and quinoa in a pot and bring it to a boil. Lower to medium-low heat and cover for 20 minutes, making sure to stir every couple of minutes. When finished, pour your quinoa in a colander to drain off excess liquid and rinse off starch with cold water. In a pan, heat coconut oil on medium-high. Add Coriander, Curry Powder and chili peppers. Stir for about 30 seconds to one minute until the chili peppers swell and coriander begins to brown.

Add Chopped Garlic and Red Onions. Stir and sauté for approximately 5 minutes until onions begin to become translucent. Add raisins, Pumpkin Seeds and cane sugar. Simmer for three more minutes or until caramelized. Lastly, add in your sea salt and cayenne pepper. Add the cooked quinoa to the pan and stir-fry for about 3 minutes. Stir in fresh squeezed lime juice and cilantro at the end (to taste).

Servings: 4-6

Buckwheat

Freedom From: Rice, Corn, Wheat and Soy.

Health Benefits: High in protein, gluten free, stabilizes blood pressure, helps regulate blood sugar, promotes heart health, has cancer-fighting antioxidants.

Flavor: Raw buckwheat has a light, nutty flavor while kasha (toasted buckwheat) has a more pronounced nutty flavor.

Consistency: Fluffy and light. When used as flour in baking it adds a fluffy, light texture to your baked goods. Buckwheat flour can be a bit tangy on its own and needs to be paired with other flours in order to balance the flavor.

RECIPE

Buckwheat Couscous
1 cup Toasted Buckwheat (Kasha)
2 cups Water
1/8 tsp. Sea Salt

DIRECTIONS:
We will use Kasha or toasted buckwheat in this recipe. Since it is already cooked, the cooking time in this recipe is very short.
Set a pot to medium low heat and add your grains.
In a separate pot, boil your water and stir in your salt. Once it comes to a boil, add it to the pot of buckwheat and let it boil fire one minute. Then cover and let simmer on low heat for 12-15 minutes. Do not stir. Remove from heat, remove the top and drain off any remaining liquid. Lightly fluff the grains with a spoon or fork, making sure not to smash the buckwheat (otherwise, the grains will become mushy). This is a delicious alternative to traditional couscous (made of wheat) or rice.

Amaranth

Freedom From: Rice, Corn, Wheat and Soy.

Health Benefits: High in proteins that are easy to digest. Gluten free. Helps strengthen bones. High in Lysine, an amino acid that many of us are deficient in and helps build muscle and produce energy. Helps regulate blood sugar, blood pressure and cholesterol. Great for heart health. High in oxalic acid (should be eaten in moderation for those with gout, kidney problems and rheumatoid arthritis).

Flavor: Amaranth has a wild, grassy flavor and is great in savory or spicy dishes.

Consistency: Grainy and crunchy

RECIPE

Amaranth Porridge
1 cup Amaranth
2 cups Water (or non-dairy Milk)
1/8 tsp. Sea Salt
2 tbsp. Cane Sugar
1 tbsp. Molasses
1/8 tsp. Ground Cloves
½ tsp. Cinnamon
1/8 tsp. Nutmeg
1 tbsp. Coconut Oil
1 cup Fresh Berries (of your choice)

DIRECTIONS:
Soak your amaranth for 12-24 hours for best results.

Bring your water or milk to a boil and add your amaranth to the pot. Let boil on medium-high heat, stirring frequently until it begins to thicken. Lower heat to medium-low and add your cane sugar, molasses, sea salt, ground cloves, cinnamon, nutmeg and coconut oil. Cook for about 15 minutes while continually stirring to make sure it does not stick. Remove from heat and let cool for 5-10 minutes. Add your berries and serve hot.

Servings: 4-5

Avocado

Freedom From: Fried and fatty foods

Health Benefits: High in potassium which helps kidney health and stabilizes energy levels. Anti-inflammatory. Full of healthy fat (oleic acid) which reduces blood pressure and helps the body absorb nutrients. Keeps you full for a long time. Assists in weight loss (due to high fiber content).

RECIPE

Avocado Salad
1 Avocado (medium ripe)
1 lime
2 tbsp. Olive Oil
1 Cucumber (diced)
1 cup Tomato (diced)
½ Onion (diced)
¼ tsp. Sea Salt

DIRECTIONS:
Cut your avocado in half and remove the seed. Using a spoon, scoop out the fruit and place on a cutting board. Dice into small pieces and add to your salad bowl. Now, dice and add your cucumber, tomato and onion to the bowl. Add fresh-squeezed lime juice, olive oil and sea salt. Stir and serve at room temperature or refrigerate and serve later.
Servings: 3-4

Beets

Freedom From: Sugar cravings

Health Benefits: Helps lower blood pressure. Removes toxins from the bloodstream and builds healthy blood cells. Boosts stamina. Anti-inflammatory. High in Vitamin C which boosts the immune system. Full of antioxidants which help prevent and fight cancer.

RECIPE

Beet Salad
1 Beetroot (boiled for 20min)
1 Lime
¼ tsp. Sea Salt
Black Pepper (to taste)
Cilantro (garnish)

DIRECTIONS:
To clean you beet thoroughly, scrub it underwater with a soft-bristle brush, making sure to remove any excess dirt. Add to a pot of boiling water and boil with the lid on for 15-20 minutes. Set aside a bowl of ice water. When the beet is done boiling, place it in the bowl of ice water and let it cool for 2-5 minutes. At this point, the skin should come off easily. Remove the skin using your hands or a paring knife. Cut the beet into paper-thin slices using a sharp knife or fruit peeler. Place your sliced beet into a bowl. Add fresh-squeezed lime juice, sea salt and black pepper. Stir and let sit for 10 minutes. Serve at room temperature or refrigerate to serve cold.
Servings: 2-4

Healthy Breakfast Alternative

Savory Oatmeal
2 cups Steel Cut Oats
4 cups Purified or Spring Water
1 tsp. Freshly Ground Rosemary
Cayenne Pepper (to taste)
½ tsp. Sea Salt
½ tsp. Paprika

Caramelized Onions:
1 White onion
2 Garlic Cloves
2 tbsp. coconut oil
½ tsp. cumin
¼ tsp. Sea Salt
¼ tsp. Paprika
1 tsp. Organic Sugar (turbinado, sucanat or regular cane sugar)
Cayenne Pepper (to taste)

DIRECTIONS:
To get the most nutrients out of this dish, soak your oaks for 12-24 hours before cooking them. On the night before you eat them, add your oats and water to a pot and bring to a boil. Remove from heat, stir in your fresh rosemary and leave covered overnight. In the morning, turn your oats onto low heat, stirring every few minutes while adding water if necessary. Dice one onion and two garlic cloves and put them to the side. Heat up your coconut oil on medium heat in a separate pan and add the minced garlic once the oil is hot. Stir for 2 minutes until it begins to brown. Then, add your onion and stir for another 5 minutes until it begins to become translucent. Add your sugar and turn the pan down to medium-low heat as you continue stirring for another 2 minutes. Add your cumin, sea salt, paprika and cayenne pepper. Your pot of oats should be finished cooking after about 15-25 minutes. Add the caramelized onion mixture to the pot of oats, mix and serve hot. Servings 2-4.

Red Lentils

Health Benefits: High in protein. Balances blood sugar. Great for long-term energy. Improves heart health. High in magnesium which improves blood flow and relaxes the muscles. Improves mood. Great alternative to beans because they are lower in phytic acid.

RECIPE

Curried Red Lentil Soup
2 cups Organic Red Lentils
3 cups Water
1 tbsp. Coconut Oil
2 tbsp. Coconut Cream
3 Garlic Cloves
1/8 tsp. Organic Cayenne Pepper
½ Lemon
½ tsp. Sea Salt
1 tbsp. Curry Powder
Or
¼ tsp. Cumin
½ tsp. Coriander
½ tsp. Turmeric

DIRECTIONS:
Soak your lentils for 12-24 hours before cooking for best results. Bring a pot of water to boil. Add lentils and lower to medium heat. Lower burner to medium heat and let simmer for 10 minutes while stirring. Lower pot to medium-low heat and cover partially (allowing some steam to release). After 5 minutes, stir in your coconut oil, coconut cream, cayenne pepper and curry powder (this can be a store bought curry powder or you may substitute by using the specified seasonings). On low heat, let it simmer with the top completely on for 3-5 minutes. Remove from heat, stir in ½ a fresh squeezed lemon and let cool.
Servings: 4-6

Savory Snack Alternative

Popcorn Style Rice Cakes
These are a great replacement for popcorn and can be a great snack when watching a movie or entertaining guests.

5 Rice Cakes (organic brown rice or wild rice based)
3 tbsp. Extra Virgin Olive Oil
¼ tsp. Sea Salt
1 tsp. Onion Powder
1 tsp. Dried Dill Weed
¼ tsp. Curry Powder
½ tsp. Sumac or Dried Lime (ground)

DIRECTIONS:
Warm up olive oil on low heat in a large pan or wok. Break up your rice cakes in a bowl until the pieces are about the size of popped popcorn. Add your rice cakes to the pan, stirring until they are completely covered in olive oil. Evenly sprinkle your seasonings over the entire pan, making sure to not put too much in one place. Stir mixture until the seasonings are covering all of the pieces. Pour into a bowl and serve warm.

Sweet Potatoes

There are many types of sweet potatoes including traditional orange, white (Japanese/Korean) and purple. All are packed with nutrients with purple sweet potatoes being the highest in health benefits.

Health Benefits: Reduce inflammation. Boost the immune system. Slow the aging process. High in potassium and help replenish energy. Balance blood sugar levels. High in beta-carotenes (vitamin A) which support healthy eyes. Full of cancer-fighting nutrients and antioxidants.

Savory Sweet Potatoes
There are a great alternative to traditional baked potatoes or french fries. Enjoy them as a finger food, light snack or side dish to accompany a meal.

3 Sweet Potatoes
2 tbsp. Coconut Oil
1 tbsp. Rosemary
1 tbsp. Oregano
1 tsp. Sumac
½ tsp. Sea Salt
1 tbsp. Dill Weed

DIRECTIONS:
Preheat your oven to 425°
Wash and skin your sweet potatoes. Then cut them into ¼ inch slices (about the width of your pinky finger). Grease the bottom of your baking pan with coconut oil. Place your sweet potato slices flat on the baking pan, making sure they do not overlap. Sprinkle rosemary, oregano, sumac, sea salt and dill weed on your sweet potatoes. Drizzle a bit of oil on top of each slice and place into the oven for 20-25 minutes. Remove and serve hot.
Servings: 3-5

Okra

Health Benefits: Assists with digestion. Eases ulcers. Balance blood sugar levels. Great for women's (womb) health. Helps heal sexual organs.

RECIPE

Oven Fried Okra

This recipe is a wonderful replacement for traditional deep-fried okra. It also helps preserve the healthy nutrients that okra is known for. Great when you are craving a salty, fatty snack.

3 cups Okra
2 tbsp. Coconut Oil
1 tbsp. Oregano
½ tsp. Sea Salt
1 tsp. Rosemary
1 tsp. Sumac
1 tbsp. Garlic Powder
1 tbsp. Onion Powder

DIRECTIONS
Preheat your oven to 450°
Place your coconut oil in a saucepan and set the temperature on low to warm it up. Thoroughly wash the okra and pat dry with a towel to make sure no water remains. Begin by cutting off the end of your okra and disposing of them. Then, slice them in half (long ways) and place them in a mixing bowl. Add your oil and seasonings to the bowl and stir until the okra is completely covered. Cover a cookie sheet or baking pan with aluminum foil. Pour your okra mixture onto the pan, making sure none of the pieces are overlapping. Place in oven and bake for 20 minutes or until the edges are golden brown. Remove from the oven and let them cool for 2-5 minutes. Serve warm.
Servings: 2-5

Healthy Homemade Dessert

Mango Sorbet
3 cups Frozen Mango Chunks
½ cup Coconut Milk/Cream
2 tbsp. Raw Honey

DIRECTIONS
With this recipe, you can buy frozen mango chunks or dice up a couple fresh mangoes and freeze them overnight.
Place your coconut milk and raw honey in a blender or food processor. Blend the mixture for 5 seconds so that the ingredients are mixed thoroughly. Add you mango chunks and pulse the blender (or food processor) until the mixture is smooth and no bits of frozen pieces are remaining. Serve immediately or store in the freezer and blend again when it is ready to be served.
Servings: 2-3

WORDS OF WISDOM

Switch it up!

Do not eat the same thing every day! Change up your meals every few days. The last thing you want to do is get sick of eating something you used to enjoy because it was all you ate day in and day out. Spice it up! Rotate your meals on a weekly basis. You can even plan ahead and make yourself a weekly menu that changes every day. Add more variety into your diet and your body will thank you for it.

What's in Your Toolbox?

A few things to invest in & why

While we are on our journey to improving our lifestyle though healthy eating, we want to get our "toolbox" in order. Below are a few tools you may want to invest in, and why:

Aside from taking supplements, a great way to step it up and get cancer fighting, anti-aging nutrients into the body is through drinking fresh juices and smoothies daily.

Juicer - Juicing Greens are an amazing way to immediately boost energy, mental focus, improve breathing, improve eyesight, curb cravings and supply the body with nutrients. Juicing is often used for medicinal purposes. Through juicing, these nutrients are delivered directly into the bloodstream and give immediate results. (COST: $40 - $300)

Blender - Like juicing, making smoothies by blending is a great way to supply the body with nutrients. The difference here is that we will stay full for a longer period of time and the nutrients take more time to get distributed throughout the body. This is good if we need something to hold us over before having a meal. (COST: $50 - $700)

*When blending or juicing, drink at least two 16-ounce glasses of water afterwards (within 30 minutes). Juicing, especially, can dehydrate the system and this will help hydrate the system and flush out any toxins that are moving out due to the nutrients we have just introduced into our system.

Here are some examples of juicing certain foods to help heal the body:
- Cucumber cleanses and balances the kidneys.
- Lemon flushes the liver.
- Ginger is anti-inflammatory and relieves allergies as well as indigestion.

In smoothies:
- The antioxidants in strawberries, blueberries and raspberries assist in reproductive health.
- The fiber in apples promote healthy bowel movements.
- The enzymes in papaya helps with digestion.

Food Processor - These machines do what blenders cannot. They break down ingredients without needing to add a lot of liquid. This allows you to make dishes like raw and vegan Brownies, sunflower seed burgers, homemade sorbets, quick chopped salads and more. We can even take whole grains and grind them into flour with these.

Herb Grinder - Buy herbs and spices whole and grind them into a powder right before you add them into your food. This not only allows us to get the most medicinal properties we can out of our spices, it makes them much more flavorful and aromatic.

Dehydrator - Make our own dried fruit, raw flaxseed crackers, raw sunflower seed burgers and more. These things suck the water out of your food so that they can remain solid without baking. This can keep us from cooking the life out of certain foods while still getting that solid, crunchy or chewy texture that you like.

Protein is Overrated

Why your protein shake may be unnecessary

Protein is made up of something called Amino-Acids. When we eat protein-rich foods (such as meat and grains), our bodies have to break those amino acids apart and reconstruct them in the body so that they can be used to build our tissue, blood cells, bones and more. These amino acids each have different effects on the body and are necessary to help the body perform different functions depending on the amino acid. This actually takes more work than simply taking in the amino acids themselves, which do not have to be broken down by the stomach, only reconstructed.

These amino acids are readily available through a multitude of fruits, vegetables, seeds, nuts and grains. There is a great deal of hype about protein, but amino acids are the building blocks of protein. There are nine essential amino acids that the body needs to function properly. Therefore, it is more important to focus on getting enough of all the necessary amino acids in your diet than protein. Protein is simply a by-product of this. You will get this balance by eating the way you naturally eat, though a balanced, plant based diet.

For example, in one day, I may have a strawberry smoothie with almond milk for breakfast, a big spinach salad with tomato and avocado for lunch, and lentil soup with a cucumber salad for dinner. In one day, I have gotten all of my essential amino acids along with the other calories, vitamins and minerals that are necessary to function as a working performing artist and travelling health-coach. I did this without having to combine different foods in one meal to create what people call "complete proteins." (such as combining beans with rice). This is a myth that was debunked in the 1950's.

The idea that plant based foods were deficient in essential amino-acids is based on studies of growing rats in the early 1900's, no humans. This ended up not being the case for humans, since we have different dietary requirements. In 1952, scientists found that all the essential amino acids could be found in many unprocessed plant foods, without food combining. In 1971, a sociologist by the name of Francis Moore Lappe wrote her bestselling book called "Diet for a Small Planet" which stated that plant foods do not have all the necessary amino acids. This was based off the false information from the early 1900's. In 1991, she recanted the statement saying that she only stated this because she was trying get more people to eat more meat in order to end world hunger (since many countries were experiencing famine due to a low amount of crops).

So, why all the hype about meat and protein? When we look at the numbers, the American RDA (Recommended Dietary Allowance) was much higher than the WHO (World Health Organization) which sets the standards for the entire world. The reality is that there is a surplus of money in the protein and meat business. Look at how many places you go and see protein powders, bars and beverages stocked on the shelves in grocery and health food stores alike. If companies were to let us know that we were already getting enough protein through eating what we eat naturally, (even on a plant based diet) then they would be out of business.

In 2001, the Nutrition Committee of the American Heart Association wrote in a medical journal that plant foods are incomplete proteins because they are missing one of more essential amino acids. This was based off of false information that had already been recanted Francis Moore Lappe and other nutrition scientists. However, in 2002, medical doctor and author John McDougall wrote to the editor, pointing out the mistake. Against the odds, they disregarded his advice and decided not to correct their mistake. This is why we hear most nutritionists and dieticians hold fast to the idea that plant foods will not give us the protein we need to sustain life. This is simply because it was written by a credible source in an official medical journal.

The WHO standards for how much protein you need a day (for adult men and women ages 18 and over) goes by 0.83 grams of protein for every kilogram that you weigh. For measurement sake, I have converted this chart from kilograms into pounds (since most of us in the United States use pounds as our measurement of weight, not kilograms).

Approximate Body Weight (lbs.)	Safe Level of Protein Intake (grams)
88	33
99	37
110	42
121	46
132	50
143	54
154	58
165	62
176	66

Protein and amino acid requirements in human nutrition
Report of a joint FAO/WHO/UNU expert consultation (WHO Technical Report Series 935), 2007, **Authors:**
World Health Organization, Food and Agriculture Organization of the United Nations, United Nations University

So, if we are around 132 pounds, then we should be getting about 50 grams of protein a day. If we weigh 93 pounds, then we should be getting around 35 grams of protein in our diets and so and so forth.

Another way to do this is to pick up a calculator and divide our weight (in pounds) by 2.2 (there a 2.2 lbs. in a kilogram) and multiply that amount by .83 to figure out how much protein we should be getting in a day. For example: I weigh 125 lbs. So, 125 ÷ 2.2 is 56.8. I take this amount (56.8) and multiply it by .83. This comes out to about a total of 47. This means I should be consuming around 47 grams of protein per day; which I am, simply by eating 3 meals a day without meat or protein supplements.

Formula:

Your weight (in lbs) ÷ **2.2** = X
Multiply (X) by **.83**
Total = recommended daily protein intake (in grams)

Example:

125 lbs. ÷ **2.2** = 56.8
56.8 × **.83** = 47
47g = recommended daily protein intake

For those who are physically active (especially athletes) or trying to build muscle mass, an increase in how many calories you consume will do the trick. Calories exist in many plant based foods, especially those high in carbohydrates including grains, fruits and starchy vegetables. No need for meat and potatoes to get to your ideal weight.

To gain muscle, simply eat more properly cooked grains as well as fresh fruits and vegetables. If we are exercising often, eat more fruit! Fruit is full of carbohydrates which will replenish our muscles and the rest of the body with the nutrients it needs.

If we are trying to lose weight, we may be able to lower our caloric intake, however, we need to continue to get the necessary amino acids and protein required for our weight in order to continue functioning properly. This will not stop us from gaining weight. As we cleanse and continue to change our lifestyle on a plant based diet, we will naturally lose excess fat as our bodies continues to get back to its naturally state.

Our bodies can only process so much protein per day. When we take in too much protein, the body does its best to excrete it through our sweat, urine and feces. Many of us are getting too much protein. When we take in 3-4 times (or more) of the recommended protein intake per day, we become at risk for many diseases. Too much protein puts stress on the kidneys and heart and can lead to dehydration as well as vitamin and mineral deficiencies.

There are now online applications that we can look up that will help us track our nutrition intake simply by entering everything we eat in a day (for example: *www.crononmeter.com)*. We may be surprised to find that we are getting more protein in our daily diets than we think, without protein supplements. If we find that we are deficient in a specific amino acid after mapping out our daily meals, research which plant based foods are high in that amino acid.

For example, parsley, spirulina (seaweed), chives, lentils and sweet green peppers are high in lysine, an essential amino acid that builds protein in the body. These foods are also high in other amino acids as well as enzymes, minerals and vitamins that help protein-synthesis in the body. Contrary to popular belief, eating meat and beans is not the only way you can reach your daily protein requirement. All fruits and vegetables are full of readily available proteins and amino acids. For example, two cups of cooked asparagus contains about 8 grams of protein. After a day of eating full meals, we will have all of the essential amino acids needed to meet our daily requirement.

The Replacement Diet

Don't waste it, replace it!

The reason most diets fail and are short-lived is because we remove things from our diets and lifestyles that we crave. These cravings only lower the quality of our lives and can actually lead to deficiencies and more health problems. Afterwards, we are left with a void and are looking for ways to fill that void. The best way we know how is to simply go back to what we are used to. This is what we call a "relapse." However, when we *replace* what we have removed with something even better, we feel better and no longer feel that void. This is what I like to call, "The Replacement Diet."

The key here is not elimination, but replacement. If we do not replace what you have removed from your life with something better, we will simply have an empty space where it used to be and you will eventually go back to what you know. We will be going over what to get rid of and how to replace it with other things we will learn to love.

WORDS OF WISDOM

"I can eat it, but I do not want it."

When we have a craving, or see something that we know we want to have but should not, we have to change our mindset and speech pattern from *"I want it but I cannot eat it"* to *"I can eat it, but I do not want it.* Why do this? The first phrase takes power away from us while the second one puts the power in our hands. The ball is in our court here. Remember that we are not taking things away from ourselves. We are giving ourselves a choice to feel and look better. When we are slowly reprogramming your mind and body to have better habits, certain experiences can make us feel like we are limiting ourselves. This is why it is important to focus on the truth. We can eat whatever we want, but we do not want it because it makes us feel bad. This is power. We can allow ourselves to feel empowered because we can finally make the choice to better ourselves and heal our families through making better choices. Not to mention, when it comes to good food, there are more options out there than we usually limit ourselves to. All it takes is a little more digging.

The "Lose It" List

How to create your personal action plan

The following is a list of ingredients that keep us in culinary bondage. Refer to the chapter on "Culinary Bondage" on page 91 for more details:

- Corn
- Wheat
- Soy
- Red Meat
- White Meat
- Fish
- Rice
- Sugar
- Honey
- Eggs
- Fried Foods
- Salty Snacks
- Dairy
- Caffeine
- Coffee
- Carbonated Beverages
- White Potatoes
- Fast Food
- Bananas
- Pasteurized Juice
- Tap Water
- Artificial Food Coloring
- Artificial Preservatives
- Artificial Flavors
- Unhealthy Cooking Oils
- Peanuts
- Alcohol
- Sulfured Dried Fruit

In order to shift into a lifestyle of eating healthily, it is helpful to create a program for ourselves. This is done by creating something called the "Lose It" list. To complete this list, you will need three things:

1.) A Journal.
2.) An open mind.
3.) The will to learn and grow.

First, start by leaving the first page of your journal blank and flipping to the second page. On the second page, brainstorm all of the things that we eat which contain ingredients on the "Lose It" list:

- Potato Chips
- Tofu
- Steak
- Hamburgers
- Ice Cream
- Soda
- Bread
- Fried Chicken
- Cheese

Second, put all of these things in order, with the first thing being the easiest to remove from our diets and the last thing being the most difficult thing to remove from our diets. Remember that this is specific to us. Only we know what we will be our greatest challenge with when it comes to removing things from our diets:

1. Tofu
2. Soda
3. Potato Chips
4. Hamburgers
5. Cheese
6. Ice Cream
7. Fried Chicken
8. Steak
9. Bread

Put this list in a visible place. For example, on the wall or refrigerator. Make copies if necessary and place them in different parts of the house. We always want to be reminded of our goals.

Starting from the top, remove one item from our diets, every three days, and replace it with a healthy option of our choice. For example:

Day 1 – Remove Tofu from my diet and replace it with Millet
Day 4 – Remove Soda from my diet and replace it with Kombucha Tea
Day 7 – Remove Potato Chips from my diet and replace it with Rice Crisps
Etc...

Continue to do this until we have replaced everything on our list. This way, you are able to pace yourself and keep track of your eating habits. It is also very rewarding to see what we have accomplished along the way. Find five minutes to journal daily while taking notes of your setbacks and accomplishments. Making this list and checking things off one-by-one gives us a greater perspective of exactly what we are eating and how it affects us. Always remembering to pace ourselves and honor the process by practicing patience. We are in control of how we eat as much as we allow ourselves to be.

Fasting

Reboot your tastebuds

Most foods are naturally sweet, spicy, sour or salty. However, we are so used to adding flavor to our food that we are unable to appreciate it. Fasting is a great way to reboot our tastebuds. Fasting will help give our tastebuds a clean slate that we can taste the inherent flavor in what we eat without having to add a bunch of unnecessary added ingredients that may harm us and your body.

Below are some examples of fasts that you can go on:

- **Salt and Sugar Fast** - Completely taking added salt and sugar out of our diets
- **Additive Fast** - Abstaining from adding any seasonings, sweeteners or oils to our food. Eating food in its natural state.
- **Liquid Fast** - Great for giving our digestive system a break. Only liquid meals including soups (without chunks of food in it), juices and smoothies.
- **Juice Fast** - Only drinking fresh pressed vegetable and fruit juice as well as water
- **Raw Foods Fast** - Only eating raw fruits, vegetables, as well as sprouted nuts and seeds. No cooked food.
- **Daytime Fast** - Only eating before sunrise and after sunset
- **Whole Food, Mono Meal Fast** - Only eating food as it came out of the earth. Often uncooked, with minimal or no additives. Eating one food per meal. (e.g.: Eating a bowl of strawberries for breakfast, two cucumbers for lunch and Brussels sprouts for dinner. No other foods.)

Do not go on a fast or detox when pregnant and do not fast for over a month. We want to allow our bodies the opportunity to heal by giving it the necessary nutrients to do so. Always drink a lot of water during a fast to keep the body hydrated and toxins to remove themselves from the liver and kidneys.

Cleanses
&
Detox Programs

When to go on one and how

From the Master Cleanse to the Liver Flush detox, there are a variety of cleanses and detox programs out there that boast about getting our bodies to perfect health. These programs often give us specific step-by-step instructions on how to detoxify our entire body or part of our bodies within a short period of time. When done too frequently or at the wrong time, these things can put undue stress on the body's internal organs, eventually doing more harm than good. We must build our bodies up to cleansing for them to be most effective. The main issue I have with these types of cleanses is that after people go through them, they go right back to the way they were living and eating. However, detoxification and cleansing programs are great when used as motivating tools along our journey towards a complete lifestyle change.

When starting cleanses or detoxes, begin by cleansing the colon first. To do this, we must be drinking enough water to urinate frequently and have clear or almost clear urine. You will also want to have at least between one and three bowel movements a day. Otherwise, when we detoxify our other organs, such as our liver and kidneys, the toxins will have no way out and will simply circulate in our bloodstream, making us feel sick. We also run the risk of these toxins and impurities depositing themselves into other parts of the body, since they have no way out. Once we have unblocked our colons and intestines, our bodies will be ready for a complete cleanse.

Listening To Your Body

Paying attention to the little things and acting on them is a form of self-love. When we feel symptoms such as aches, pains, itchiness, tightness in the chest or loss of energy our bodies are telling us what state it is in. These types of reactions also tell you if you have an intolerance to something almost immediately after you eat it. This is why detoxifying the body helps. After years of eating things that hurt the body, we build up a callousness, which numbs our bodies to the discomfort we are feeling.

Carpenters and construction workers have something in common. When we look at their hands, they are rough. The skin on them is thick and calloused. After years of constant abrasions, this callousness protects them from feeling pain and discomfort while working. The same thing happens inside the body.

When we beat up our organs day after day, year after year, they become calloused. We no longer feel the uncomfortable side effects of eating the harmful foods we have been eating all our lives because our bodies have built up a defense against feeling them. Once we detox, removing the toxins from our system that were left over from years of improper eating, our bodies will get used to not having these things in our system. It will open up and relax. It becomes easier to be in tune with how the body feels at all times, empowering us to truly be at our best. Inside and out!

WORDS OF WISDOM

Trying old foods with new habits

After removing certain foods from our diet, we often become interested to see how our bodies will respond to those foods, or simply miss them so much that we cannot help ourselves. The rule of thumb is to wait until you have cleansed your body of that ingredient or food group for at least three months. Allow yourself to "dip your toe in the pool" first. Do not just dive in. In other words, do not binge. We will only feel horrible afterwards. However, if we can avoid eating it at all because we know it is not good for us, then do so.

It's a Process, Not a Diet

Honoring every step of the way

Regardless if we call ourselves a "Vegan", "Vegetarian" or "Carnivore" there is no need to feel pressured to subscribe to a label. The problem most people have with most diets of cleanses is that they are extreme. For this reason, they do not feel natural and, in turn, they do not last long. Though some of us may be able to go cold turkey when it comes to certain things we eat, most of us struggle with the idea. Even after we "successfully" go cold turkey off of eating something we know is not good for us, most of us struggle with staying the course over a long period of time. For the rest of us, the physical, mental and emotional shock we experience when it comes to going cold turkey off of a food addiction is too much. A better way to go about this is to look at this as a *process* to improve our *lifestyle* in relation to how we eat. This could take two weeks or two years.

Regardless, it is smarter to wean yourself off of a food addiction by gradually replacing it with healthier alternatives until you reach your goal. This way, we will experience long-term results. For me, it was a two year process from eating everything under the sun (except red meat) including fast food a few days a week to thriving off a plant based diet including 75% live foods (uncooked fruits and vegetables as well as sprouted nuts and grains). The goal here is consistency and sustainability, not a quick fix. We want to be healthy for life, not for two months.

I started my journey with something I called the "Elimination Diet". In order to find out what was causing my eczema, I took everything out of my diet except for rice. Then, I continued to add an ingredient on, day by day. Anytime I had a negative reaction to what I was eating, I would take note of it and remove it from my diet. Fortunately for me, I love to cook and have a knack for creativity. But, it took me years to figure out how to eat properly without having certain things in my diet. The problem with diets such as the elimination diet is that after we have stopped eating all of these things, we usually do not replace them with anything good and tasty. Then, we are left feeling a void that needs to be filled. What do we fill it with you ask? The same thing we stopped eating! This happens all the time. So, how do you avoid this? Simply, by replacing what we remove out of our eating lifestyles with something just as delicious and nutritious. This is where we have room to get creative. There are simple ways to do this that are listed in the book, however, feel free to get creative as you want. There are so many options out there and it is amazing how accessible they are.

Almost all of us are addicted to some kind of food. How many people do you know cannot have a complete day without their cup of coffee, soda, bag of chips or even a slice of pie? Are we one of those people? The truth is, most of us are. How do we know if we are addicted to something we are eating or drinking? Think about anything we may be eating regularly that may not be so good for us. Now, think about not eating or drinking it for a year. Then, commit to this idea. If we can do this, and not feel tempted to even touch whatever it may be for a year, not even a taste, congratulations! We are not human. However, if we cannot deal with that idea, without feeling a little crazy (like most of us when it comes to something we love eating/drinking), then we may be addicted to whatever it is we are eating and drinking.

The purpose of this book is not to say that everything we eat is bad and that we need to stop it *right now*. It is to serve as a guide to empower others to change their eating habits over time by replacing them with healthier eating habits. Little by little. Day by day.

WORDS OF WISDOM

The slip-up cure

When we slip up and eat something we are trying to take out of our diets (and we all do, because we are human) take these steps:

1. Stop, reassess, and honor where we are emotionally.
2. Take the experience as a lesson.
3. Remember how much we want to reach our goals and use this as motivation to keep going.

We all want to feel good and we all deserve to feel good. So we must cut ourselves some slack. Tomorrow is another day!

Living Situations

Eating well no matter where you live

When we do not live by ourselves, and are sharing our space with others, things can get tricky. Especially if the other people do not fully support our healthy lifestyle or eat the same way we do.

One of the most difficult places to eat healthy is when living in a college dorm. As we are surrounded by fast food and fried food. Most of this food only fills us up for the moment, but we are left feeling tired because we are not getting the nutrients we need. So, most of us supplement this with caffeinated drinks, however, these do not really help us study for an exam as much as they give you "the jitters". Not to mention, we most likely do not have access to a cooking facility and we are sharing our space with someone else.

Solutions:
- Get an electric griddle (if the school allows it).

- Electric Kettle to boil water (and other liquids) to make hot drinks or quick soups.
- Invest in a small blender for energy-boosting and long lasting smoothies.
- Get a table and cutting board for preparing live foods such as salads.
- Purchase a used mini fridge to store all of pre-made meals for later use.
- Stock up on tupperware, travel mugs, snack bags and plastic utensils, prep meals and take these in a bag to eat in a pinch.

Keep this in mind, if you are living in a shared apartment or multigenerational home. These tools can be used to your benefit as well.

Microwaves

More than a quick fix

Lose the microwave. Do not touch it. Even in a pinch. It is healthier to have our food cold than it is to use one of these things. First of all, they zap almost all of the nutrients out of your food. Sometimes, this is done to the point where our bodies does not even register it as food and has trouble digesting it. Then, it introduces harmful radiation to your home or office. Try to avoid these machines as much as possible, no matter how convenient it may be. Do a quick online search for the harmful effects of long-term microwave use on our health. When in doubt, go the cooking route.

Occupational Hazard

Eating well no matter where your work

Many of us have occupations where we travel and are out of the house quite often. Truck Drivers, Lawyers and Performing Artists all have it tough when it comes to having the time to get access to healthy and affordable food. We usually do not have the time (or energy) to prepare food at home and we end up eating what is convenient (and usually unhealthy). I would know. I have been a touring performing artist for over 10 years. The best advice I could give you are these two gems:

1.) **Preparation**: Buy some good tupperware, a leak-resistant thermos, a bunch of napkins and take your utensils from home. If we have early mornings, prep our food the night before so we can simply throw it together in the morning. This may involve, chopping veggies and even par-boiling some foods so they take less time in the morning. Choose meals that do not necessarily need to be heated up, like salads and grains. This way we will not be tempted to use a microwave. We can also pack snack bags of dried fruit, nuts, fresh fruits or raw vegetables (I have learned to love carrots and cucumbers, chopped and lightly seasoned). For our juices or smoothies, we can pre-wash and chop our fruits or vegetables as well. All we have to do in the morning is blend/juice and throw it in our thermos!

2.) **Research**: Since we live in the information age, we can look almost anything up on the internet. We can search for places that cater to our healthy-eating needs. Look at their online menu and inventory, make a few phone calls and, "bam!" We have a list of places we can fall back on when we are on the run.

WORDS OF WISDOM

Eating light

Snacking is good for us! Five small meals a day is better than 1-2 heavy meals a day. It is a good practice to carry some fruit or a bag of nuts with us for when we get hungry. This helps boost our energy and metabolism. We will feel lighter and have more energy throughout the day.

Eating Out

How to find healthy food on the go

If we are out and want to have a good time, or simply do not feel like cooking at home, there are many options out there. We tend to limit ourselves to the same diners, restaurants and cafes. However, there is a world of flavor out there, and it is often right in our cities! Aside from our traditional soup and salad shops or vegan/vegetarian restaurants, the world of international cuisine has many options in regards to healthy eating. Many of these countries have vegetarian, vegan, soy free and wheat free options. Below are a few examples of international cuisines along with their qualities. Take the time to search for these types of restaurants in your area. Dive into a new culture and ask the waiter for the most authentic dishes you can get. Your taste buds will thank you!

- **Thai, Vietnamese, Malaysian, Chinese Cuisine** – Rice noodle based dishes. Curries. Soups.
- **Nepali, Indian Cuisine** – Curries. Rice and vegetable dishes. Rice and lentil-based breads.
- **Ethiopian, Eritrean Cuisine** - Injera (made of Teff, which serves as the base of all dishes), spicy vegetable options.
- **Persian, Greek, Moroccan, Turkish Cuisine** – Bean-based dishes. Fresh and grilled vegetables. Curries.

246

Shopping Around

Where to get good food

We may be wondering how to find the ingredients that are listed in this book. There are three main places where we can get healthy food:

Farmers Market: If we can find a farmers market nearby, this is a great option for local produce and farm-raised meat. The wonderful thing about farmers markets is that everything they sell is almost always in season and you can actually talk to the people who work with the farm. This means that we are directly connected to the source of our food (as opposed to allowing the grocery store to be the middle-man). This gives a great advantage to you (the customer) when it comes to knowing where your food comes from and how it was treated. Furthermore, some farmers markets are seasonal and we may only see them in the warmer months when crops are ripe.

Health Food Store: Many cities have local health food stores. Some of these stores are small and some are as big as shopping malls. These are also great places to shop and most of the employees will be able to give us advice on where to get what we are looking for (even outside of the store). Thus, health food stores are almost always tied into a community of conscious, healthy eating people. This is a great way to get connected with others who will support our healthy lifestyle.

Online: The internet has opened up the world to us in ways that were unimaginable a few years ago. If we cannot find any of the places listed above by asking people in your community or searching the internet, then you can always shop online. Today, there are hundreds of online stores, which specialize in selling healthy foods at affordable prices. Combining your local shopping with online shopping is often a good strategy here.

Breaking the bank?
A basic plant based diet is actually quite affordable (quality cuts of meat cost more than organic fruits and vegetables). When it comes to healthy eating, a gourmet raw foods diet is more costly than a simple plant based diet. Keep it basic! When we cook less (as opposed to cooking the life out of something), we get more out of our food. This is because we are getting more nutrients out of what we eat. Stick to this advice and you will find that you will get full by eating less, buying less and spending less.

WORDS OF WISDOM

The "health food" phase

"Health Food" is not always healthy. Just because it is in a Health Food Store does not mean that it is good for us either. Be wary of the labels we put on certain types of foods and we have to decipher for ourselves what is best for us.

The "Food Desert" Epidemic

One of the biggest challenges our people face today is a lack of places to get healthy food. Food Deserts are areas in the country where there are not enough resources to buy things such as fresh and organic produce. These cities and neighborhoods are filled with liquor stores, corner stores and fast food restaurants. These places are set up as the only places in the area to get a quick bite or to grab something to drink. The issue is that what these places are feeding us is killing us and we have nothing else in the area to balance the situation. This way, we keep getting sick and the hospitals and clinics continue to admit us without offering a healthier solution.

So, what is the solution? One of the best ways is to order online. Write a letter to your local grocery store requesting fresh, organic options and healthier brands. Seek out and support a local garden or farm or even start one. One of the reasons that these places do not exist in certain areas is because they think they will not get enough customers in order to make enough money. Show that there is an interest by signing a petition for a health food chain to be opened in the neighborhood or in one nearby. We have to be the change that we want to see. It is key to educate people in our circles about healthy eating by leading through example. We never know what we can accomplish until we try.

"What is well rooted cannot be pulled up. What is firmly grasped will not slip loose. It will be honoured from generation to generation."

-Lao Tzu

Suggested Reading

Wheat Belly: Lose the Wheat, Lose the Weight, and Find Your Path Back to Health by William Davis

The Whole Soy Story: The Dark Side of America's Favorite Health Food by Kaayla T. Daniel

Food Combining (In a Nutshell) by Kathryn Marsden

Heal Your Body by Louise Hay

Eat Right for 4 Your Type: Complete Blood Type Encyclopedia by Peter D'Adamo

The Everything Anti-Inflammation Diet Book by Karlyn Grimes

Water: For Health, for Healing, for Life: You're Not Sick, You're Thirsty! by F. Batmanghelidj

Heal Thyself for Health and Longevity by Queen Afua

The City of Wellness: Restoring Your Health Through the Seven Kitchens of Consciousness by Queen Afua

The Kemetic Diet: Food For Body, Mind and Soul, A Holistic Health Guide Based on Ancient Egyptian Medical Teachings by Muata Ashby

For more information on recipes, detox programs and workshops, join the movement at:

www.BreakingFoodChains.com

Questions, comments or suggestions?

Please email them to

info@breakingfoodchains.com

Made in the USA
Charleston, SC
04 October 2016